Stand UP, Stand OUT, Stand STRONG

A 30-Day Guide to Navigate Life

When the SHIFT Hits the Fan

Sue Dumais

Published by Heart Led Living Publishing, December, 2018
ISBN: 9780995813045

Editor: Nina Shoroplova
Typeset: Greg Salisbury
Cover Design: Judith Mazari
Cover Digital Painting: Sarah Scheifele
Sue Dumais's Portrait Photographer: Adrienne Thiessen of
        Gemini Visuals Creative Photography

The book is a gift for everyone, everywhere, all at once.

Testimonials

"One thing I found absolutely incredible about Sue is her intuition and powerful ability to have that resonate for my deepest growth. Sue is particularly amazing at reminding me what is soul inspired and what is not, and creating the space to be spirit led. I would highly recommend Sue to anyone looking to be more heart led in all that they are and do in the world."

Lara Kozan, Co-Founder YYoga & Nectar Juicery, Entrepreneur, Coach

"Sue is the clearest channel I have encountered and I trust her whole heartedly. She has a way of helping me to see all that life brings in a new light and to unwind my mind in a way that has transformed many situations in my life. Sue's words and teachings speak deeply to me and bring a sense of calm and clarity."

Natalie McGrorty, Intuitive Coach, Massage Therapist and Women's Health Educator

"When I reflect on the work that I have received and the work that others have received from Sue, I am always amazed. She has an ability to take you further into yourself, into a place where you have not necessarily realized or seen before. Sue has opened me up, allowing me to feel my body more, my emotions more and my heart more. She has an ability to help you realize what you need to heal and let go of and is a mastermind when it comes to the heart connection and universal life."

Kelly Van Unen, Best-Selling Author, Intuitive Coach, Inside Out Life Consultant

"The depth of healing and shifts in perspective that take place when working with Sue is unparalleled."
Diana Calvo, Best-Selling Author, Former Corporate Executive, Life Transition Coach

"Sue Dumais will challenge you to stand in your power, get out of your comfort zone and stand up for what you believe in. Sue's message comes from her heart. It will stop you from running and make you face the truth of who you are, and that will set you free."
Les Brown, World Renowned Motivational Speaker, Speech Coach, Author

"Mastery is what comes to mind when I think about Sue Dumais as a coach and intuitive healer. Through her masterful art I have become more confident in trusting, listening and being guided by my intuition, this has provided me with substantial growth personally and professionally. "
Kate Muker, Conscious Divas Founder, Entrepreneur, Speaker

Acknowledgements

My gratitude runs deep and it feels as though my heart has grown two sizes in the process of writing this book. So many miracles. So much support. So much love.

Thank you to my husband and two children for their unwavering support as they held down the fort at home so I could spend three weeks in Turks and Caicos to create space for this book to come to fruition. Your love, encouragement, and patience is deeply appreciated.

Thank you to my publisher and writing coach, Julie Salisbury, for once again guiding and loving me through the process of getting the words from my heart onto the pages of this book.

Thank you to my editor, Nina Shoroplova, for your gentle guidance and master wordsmithing skills to bring this book to the world.

Thank you to my membership and program coordinator, friend, and my right hand, Kimberly Shuttleworth, for your endless support and encouragement. You are one of my greatest cheerleaders.

Thank you to my community, my Heart Led Living family, and all the beautiful souls and light leaders who have joined our Heart YES Movement. Your courage, determination, and willingness to heal and shine brightly in this world are palpable and will inspire many. You have renewed my faith in humanity and continue to fuel my passion to impact change and heal the world.

And I am deeply grateful to you for picking up this book and being open to trying on another perspective. Thank you for being curious. Thank you for being willing. Thank you for being you. The world needs you now more than ever. As we join our hearts and unite in love we become a powerful force for change.

Thank you from the depths of my heart and soul.

Heart hugs,

Sue Dumais

Contents

Introduction

It is clear the world is changing. Many people believe things are getting worse and we are going backwards but the truth is, everything is getting uncovered and brought out into the open. This is the good news. Anything that remains hidden won't change and can't be healed.

The question most people want answered is, how do we navigate this shift that is occurring on our planet? How can we meet the fear, judgment, hatred, anger, and violence without fighting against it and adding more fear?

As I reflect on what it took to bring this book to life, I am in awe of the process. I practically wrote it with my eyes closed. I had no idea of what each chapter topic would be until it was finished. The chapters came out in sound bites, often in the wee hours of the morning. I had no idea what I was writing until the words stopped flowing through my fingers and I would read what I wrote. Whenever I felt resistance or went into my head to figure it out, I would stop and walk away. I was practising deep trust and writing with blind faith.

All I knew for sure was that this book needed to be written at this time. I knew in my heart that there are people waiting for this message and many are calling for some form of a guide to help them navigate this incredibly challenging shift that is happening on our planet. Yes, it is incredibly challenging and it is literally shaking the ground beneath our feet. At the same time, it is waking us all up and exposing some deep darkness that has remained hidden for a long time. Everything is being brought into the light of awareness so we can heal deeply and collectively.

This book is designed to challenge our programmed thinking minds. The messages may not be what we want to hear, but I guarantee they are what we need to hear in order to unwind our minds and open our hearts. This thirty-day guide will shake us up to wake us up to a new way of being in relationship with each other.

This global shift is necessary. It is essential. It is timely. If we are to change what is no longer working so we can evolve as a species, we must all find a way to navigate this shift and be willing to play our part. It is important to remember that everyone's part is essential.

The time is now! No more turning a blind eye. No more pretending. No more hiding. No more trying to fit in. Let's bring it all into the light of awareness and ride this wave of change and evolution so we can unite in love for each other and our planet. It is time for all of us to Stand UP, Stand OUT, and Stand STRONG.

Take my hand. Let's begin together ....

Day 1

When We Care Too Much, It Hurts

Day 1 ~
When We Care Too Much, It Hurts

Caring too much can be more harmful than helpful. The idea that we should be caring and compassionate individuals is not a new concept. We are taught at a very young age to care about others but the problem is that there is more importance placed on caring about what others think, do, and have. We are often programmed to care more about other people's lives and their opinions than our own lives and opinions.

"What will the neighbours think?"

"Stop doing that—everyone is watching."

We learn to care so much that we are in constant judgment or fear of judgment, judging whether others are good or bad, rich or poor, kind or mean, healthy or unhealthy; judging whether they like us or not and whether they approve of what we are doing or not doing. Caring more about others becomes a distraction from caring about ourselves and it also opens us up to deep hurt and more harm than good.

When I was knee-deep into the fitness and wellness industry, I was a sponge for knowledge. I was constantly taking courses, reading books, and studying research. I was consumed with finding out how the body works and what makes it tick. I was addicted to health and sharing that message with others. It fed my childhood desire to save the world. In truth, it wasn't just a strong desire—it became my responsibility. In other words, I made it my mission, my responsibility. It was on my shoulders to save the world and everyone in it, including the animals. Just a small burden to bear!

When people were interested in what I had to teach them, it was easy, fulfilling, and I felt a deep sense of purpose and impact. But my desire to save the world wasn't just for those who were interested or ready to be saved. I wanted to help EVERYONE whether they wanted help or not. I thought if I could just teach them what I knew they would see how important it was and they would make the changes they needed to make to become healthy. I would give advice when it wasn't welcome. I would invest much time and energy trying to make others see the truth. I wanted them to "get it" so badly it consumed me. My love for them was fierce and I would stop at nothing.

I cared so much that if they didn't change, I felt responsible. I cared so much that I became attached to whether they changed or not. I cared so much that I became attached to them taking the information and doing something with it. I cared so much that I became anxious and I worried about others constantly. I cared so much that I alienated some people in my life because I just wanted so badly for them to be healthy, happy, and live a long life. When they didn't "get it" or I wasn't able to help them, I was devastated. I carried them with me as one of my failures. I had failed to help them. I had failed to help them see. I had failed to change their mind. I had failed. I started to realize that caring too much was a heavy burden full of disappointment and suffering.

I remember shortly after I healed from cancer, I became obsessively worried about my family's health. I was eating super clean food with no sugar, no wheat, no gluten, and no dairy;

I was eating mostly organic; I was green juicing every day. After being diagnosed with a genetic liver disorder, I was more aware of what I put in my mouth and how it would affect my health. My worry started to grow exponentially when I would compare how I was eating to how my husband and kids were eating. They had already said my diet was too extreme for them, but my fear kept growing and I felt heavy and responsible for keeping them healthy and safe. At the same time, I felt out of control because I couldn't control everything they put in their mouths and their resistance to eating my way was strong. They ate mostly healthfully, but my fear-filled mind had me convinced it wasn't healthy enough.

One morning in meditation I started to feel a huge layer of fear rising up around the health of my husband. He was stressed at work, he had gained some weight, and I kept being pointed to his heart. I felt this huge mountain of responsibility for keeping him healthy. I had a painful vision of him dying; and of me standing over his grave with a "guilty" sign strung around my neck. Tears streamed down my cheeks as though a faucet were pouring uncontrollably. I felt responsible for his health and I believed that if he died it would be all my fault. I would be responsible for his death because I hadn't been able to convince him to change his ways. The burden was unbearable and it cracked my heart open.

My ego mind had convinced me I was responsible for the health of my family because I bought the groceries. So if something would have happened to them, it would have been all my fault. Later that night, I shared my vision with my husband and told him the burden I was carrying. I explained how if he died it would be all my fault. His words were such a gift as they landed in a way that shifted everything for me. He said, "You are not responsible for me or anyone else's health.

My health choices are my health choices, not yours."

I suddenly saw an opening in my mind and the terrifying grip of fear let go; a huge sense of relief washed over me. I couldn't force them to eat a certain way. Trust me—I had tried and it hadn't worked. Forcing them is not empowering them. It is not up to me; it is up to them. They must make the choice for themselves.

I felt a freedom I never felt before. It was as though I let go of a lifetime of attachment to the choices others make or don't make. It is not up to me. I can empower them with knowledge but ultimately they need to feel empowered by making their own choices. I can show up and play my part but the rest is not up to me. It is like that old saying, "You can lead a horse to water, but you cannot make it drink." In my life and in my home, I lead by example. I buy healthy foods and make healthy meals, but my family doesn't need to eat a hundred percent healthy all the time unless they want to. I have processed my fears, let go of my attachments around their health, and I accept their choices. I have also slowly let go of my judgments about their choices and freed them to empower themselves. I still make decisions for my son around food, only because he would eat sugar all day long if I let him. The difference is when I do say no or yes to certain foods, it is now coming from a place of love not paralyzing fear and control disguised as caring.

We are programmed to care so much that we want to help, give advice, fix, change, and make right what we think is wrong in other people's lives. The Truth is that other people's lives are none of our business, but we make them our business and that can come at a great sacrifice and much suffering.

Let's take a look at the news for a moment. Do you feel better or worse after watching, reading, or listening to the news? I have come to believe that CNN stands for "constant negative news." We are bombarded with images and stories that build fear and make us feel guilty for what we have, bad for what we don't, and even worse for others. When we care so much that we feel sick to our stomach or we develop chronic anxiety about everything that is going wrong in the world, we are not helping; we are causing more harm. We are causing more harm to our own well-being, but we are also adding more fear to an already fear-filled world.

~

Caring for others in the form of worry is the same as sprinkling them with fear.

~

I used to believe that caring showed others that I loved them. People don't need you to care in the form of worry. That is the same as sprinkling them with fear. People want to feel loved, and caring too much is not an expression of love: it is an expression of fear. So not only are we adding more fear to the pot, we are causing more suffering inside our own mind as we learn to chronically fret and worry about others. That is not loving to others or ourselves.

The world doesn't need more fear and neither do we. What we all need is more authentic genuine expressions of love sprinkled with empathy and compassion. Empathy calls us to imagine how they must be feeling and loving them in spite of those feelings. It is about being present for them to express and share how they feel without our judging them or trying to fix them or change how they feel. Just loving them in that moment and holding space for them to feel fully so they can heal is enough.

~

*Meeting their fear with your unconditional love and being
a compassionate witness allows them to feel heard, seen, and
understood and at the same time allows us to hold the high
note and stand strong in the energy of love.*

~

Instead we are taught to sympathize with others and their situations, but sympathy is about feeling sorry for them. People don't need us to feel sorry for them and it only leaves us feeling bad at the same time. Meeting them in the fear with our own fear is not helpful. Meeting their fear with your unconditional love and being a compassionate witness allows them to feel heard, seen, and understood and at the same time allows us to hold the high note and stand strong in the energy of love.

Today, I do my best to see everyone through the lens of love. I honour where they are and accept that some are willing to heal and some are not. The difference from the way I used to be is I now see everyone as capable. I see everyone's potential and I focus on that without attachment. I know that beyond their fear is all the love they could ever need or ever ask for. We all have access to that love. Some will turn toward the love and say YES and others will turn away from it and say no. I accept and honour them either way. I love them just the same. Now that doesn't mean I devote my time and energy trying to help them all. I simply love them and I trust my heart to lead me. I will either be guided to help them or I won't.

My responsibility is not to save the world any more, but to support those I am meant to support and free everyone else to live their life. I trust that if someone is meant to work with me, they will find their way back or they will find someone else who is. The pressure is off my shoulders because I took it off.

The burden is no longer mine to carry because I put it down. I no longer care too much, but I have learned to love deeply without attachment and that has been the biggest gift I could have ever given myself and the world.

Day 2

We Are More Connected Than We Are Separate

Day 2 ~
We Are More Connected Than
We Are Separate

Knowing we are connected to others is not a radical idea; it is something that many people experience on a daily basis without realizing it. The idea of oneness has been talked about forever, but the experience of oneness seems to be fleeting or it happens without people knowing it.

Just for fun, imagine your mind is wide open to trying on a different perspective. Be open and curious at the same time, so you can place judgment aside and see what happens with this idea as it comes into your awareness. All I am asking is that you let go of everything you think you know and be wide open to another perspective, even if it is just while you are reading this.

The biggest block to new ideas is that we already think we know what we don't know. What if everything we thought we knew wasn't true?

What if the world we see is limited by the lens we are programmed to look through?

What if everything we think we see in front of us is just an illusion created and programmed by our minds?

What if it was only our own judgments that make us believe we are separate from everyone and everything?

When I was a child I had a very painful internal environment. My mind was often a thought storm of fear, worry, and anxiety.

The only time I felt some peace of mind was when I was in nature. As a child I was fascinated with any and all things natural—forests, trees, leaves, stones, rocks, shells, sand, mud, flowers, plants, insects, animals, lakes, streams, rivers, frogs especially tadpoles—essentially any and all things in nature. Even when I felt disconnected from everything including my sense of self, I could enter a forest or sit by a lake and I would feel an instant connection with nature. My mind became still and I experienced a sense of peace.

~

I could enter a forest or sit by a lake and I would feel an instant connection with nature.

~

My senses were so heightened when I was in nature that I could find the tiniest things and they would bring me joy. I remember finding a tiny frog the size of my thumb nail. When I showed others they asked, "How did you ever find something so small?" and my answer was, "How could you not see it?" It was as though I had magnified x-ray vision in nature. I could see and appreciate all the little details in everything I found. I would collect rocks and shells. I would even hold onto different pieces of driftwood that resembled shapes of animals; well, they did through my eyes.

Every summer we stayed with my grandparents at their cottage on a lake in Northern Ontario. I would ride my bike along the road to this one path through the forest that led to a huge rock at the edge of the lake. The only way to get there was by this path or by boat. As a child, it seemed like a massive rock. Everything was so quiet when I went there, including my monkey mind. It was as though life slowed down and all was well in the world. I felt peace within and all around me. The rest of the world and all its problems disappeared and I was fully present to every detail and at the same time I felt deeply connected to everything.

Connecting to nature is a common way many people experience oneness. Perhaps you enjoy walking in nature or you are fascinated by the moon or the stars. Some people feel this connection when playing with a child or holding an infant. Others may experience oneness through physical intimacy or feeling the depth of love they have for someone in their life.

What creates a sense of peace within you?

What experiences are you most drawn to that bring you peace and calm?

What soothes your heart?

What calms your mind?

What gives you a sense of connection to nature or others?

We have all had experiences of oneness but most of us haven't been aware of it. Let me remind you, we are having some fun here, trying on a different perspective. It will be easy for some and mind bending for others. Remain open and curious.

On the surface, we judge that we all look different and seem separate, but if we go beyond our programmed mind and beyond what the naked eye can see, we all share a connection. From our limited human perspective, we are each separate human beings walking around this planet. There are trees, cars, mountains, oceans, and millions of other things that we see as separate from ourselves.

Let's first begin with a change in perspective. Bring an image of a leaf from a particular tree into your awareness for a moment. Notice the veins, the patterns, and the texture of the leaf. That leaf is just a leaf on its own, separate from everything else. Now imagine the leaf on a branch and the branch holding other leaves that are similar and at the same time unique. Now visualize the branch as connected to the trunk of a tree just like many other branches with many other leaves. Again all are similar and at the same time unique. Now, I invite you to change your perspective to see the whole tree with its branches, leaves, bark, and roots. Instead of seeing each part of it as separate, see the tree in all its beauty. Just by changing our perspective, we can change what we see. We can zoom in and see one leaf on the tree again, or zoom out and see the whole tree.

According to quantum physics everything is made up of energy. The denser its energy, the more solid an object appears. If you took an object and put it under one of the world's most powerful microscopes you could zoom in and start to see the workings of that object. I used to work as a Registered Veterinary Technician and I loved looking under a microscope. It opened up a whole new perspective that fascinated me. Looking at blood cells under a microscope and even analyzing stool samples for parasites were intriguing and exciting activities for me.

What if we could replace the lens in our physical eye with a microscopic lens? What if we could zoom in on objects and start to see their inner workings? What if we could zoom out and see the bigger picture like we did with the tree, but do it with the world, our solar system, our galaxy? Where does one thing separate from another? At what perspective do we begin to see just the leaf and shift to seeing the whole tree?

Now that we can see the whole tree we can appreciate that all parts of the tree contribute to the health of the entire tree. For example if one leaf became infected with a fungus, that fungus could spread and eventually impact the health of the entire tree and it might also spread to all the trees around it, impacting the entire forest.

In British Columbia, Canada, we have a mountain pine beetle that is a natural resident in the Rocky Mountains. Mountain pine beetles cause damage to pine trees throughout the province, by laying eggs under the bark and introducing a fungus that interferes with water and nutrient absorption. The pine needles on the branches dry up and turn brown as the tree dies. Our cold winters control the numbers of this insect. In the late 1990s, several warm winters allowed the population of pine beetles to skyrocket, which resulted in a loss of millions of hectares of pine trees over a period of about fifteen years. If we zoom out from one tree to a forest of trees to a province of trees we can get an idea of how the sum of the parts affects the whole.

It was the philosopher Aristotle who first coined the phrase, "The whole is greater than the sum of its parts." In other words, everything we do individually contributes to the whole of humanity. In every moment our actions and nonactions are either helping humanity or harming humanity. Intentionally or unintentionally, we are constantly contributing to the whole of humanity. Therefore, if we hold the vision of working together and we are willing to play our part, we can positively impact the world as a whole and at the same time uplift humanity.

The questions are "Can we put aside our differences and can we begin to see we are much more alike than we have been taught?" If we ask "How are we the same?" we can clearly see that we are all human and that we are all part of this world. In other words, we are a sum of all the unique parts that make up the whole of humanity and, if we zoom out, we see the whole planet and then if we zoom out further the whole galaxy and then the whole universe. So what part do you want to play? Do you wish to contribute to the problems, to be the pine beetle? Or do you wish to be part of the solution? If we each play our part, together, we can affect the change that leads to unifying us in love through connection, cooperation, and collaboration.

Day 3

Born Innocent, Programmed Guilty

Day 3 ~
Born Innocent, Programmed Guilty

We can look at a newborn baby or a baby animal and see its innocence and feel love expanding in our hearts. As young babies, we were curious and wide open to exploring the world through innocent eyes. Not only were we experiencing our own innocence, but we could see the innocence of others. We began our lives with a curious wide-open mind and a soft heart. We would observe the world around us and everyone in it without judgment or preconceived notions, because we had no preconceived filter, programming, or conditioning.

Imagine for a moment that when each of us is young, our mind is a new computer with very few programs added; it is running smoothly. As we grow, we receive programs and downloads from the world around us. Our parents, friends, family, teachers, strangers, TV, movies, radio, music, and books all contribute to the programs that begin to act like filters through which we interpret and experience our world. Up until the age of five or six, our conscious mind is unable to accept or deny these downloads. Like a sponge, the young mind takes in everything it is exposed to without question. All the programming is accepted and downloaded without our conscious choice or awareness. This becomes the filter through which we interpret the world around us.

If one of our filters is based on fear, we will filter our life through that lens of fear and our experiences in life will be fear-based. If one of our filters is based on love and compassion, we filter our life through that lens of love, and our experiences will be more loving. What we believe we perceive and what we perceive we conceive.

~

What we believe we perceive and what we perceive we conceive.

~

Our minds are programmed to fear or love. In fact in every moment, we are choosing fear or love. We are either doing this by default based on our programming or we are doing it on purpose. My programming was very much based on fear, worry, anxiety, judgment, and pain. Every experience I had growing up was filtered through this lens of fear and it created an internal hell. On the outside, I was more worried about how others would feel and my fear of being judged was strong, so I pretended to be okay. I wore a mask of a shy little girl who was okay; meanwhile on the inside, I was in excruciating emotional pain.

My mind was an intense relentless storm by the time I was six years old. I blamed myself for everything. I felt responsible for everything wrong in the world; my filter showed me a ton of evidence to prove the world was full of pain and suffering, and it was entirely my fault. I turned to self-destructive behaviours as forms of self-punishment—I struggled with substance abuse, anorexia, bulimia, and self-hatred.

At the same time as I condemned myself, I strived to make a difference in the world, partially in an effort to make up for my sins and worthlessness, but also because it was programmed

24

in my heart to be of service, to be a peacekeeper, to inspire others. The problem came when I felt I needed to pay my dues by being of selfless service to others. Yes, I did have a positive impact on the lives of others but it came at a great cost of self-sacrifice.

My self-judgment was intense. Here is a glimpse into some of my internal dialogue. Even though I have censored it a bit, it will give you a good idea of the destructive judgments that kept me imprisoned in guilt and shame for years.

"I am guilty."

"I am a worthless piece of sh…"

"I don't deserve to be happy. Actually, I don't deserve anything other than punishment."

"I will spend the rest of my life trying to make up for my inadequacies."

"I am not good enough and I will never be enough for anything or anyone."

"I hate myself and everything about me."

"Nobody loves me or even cares I am here. I might as well be dead."

After receiving counselling for my eating disorder in 1993, I realized I needed to change my thoughts in order to change my experience of life. While I couldn't control the thoughts that came into my mind, I could begin to challenge them. I remember hearing someone say that we don't need to believe all of our thoughts and, in fact, most our own thoughts are not true. That was comforting and I was determined to change my self-destructive thoughts and find some peace of mind. It has been a process of unwinding my fear-filled, critical mind and reprogramming it for love.

~

While I couldn't control the thoughts that came into my mind,
I could begin to challenge them.

~

Over the years I have created new filters and downloaded new programs. I remind myself every day to love and accept myself. I made a conscious choice for love over and over again until it began to feel easier and more natural, and my internal programming shifted from fear to love. I admit it is still a work in progress, but I align more with love than I experience fear, and when I do experience fear, I have the tools and awareness to shift my thoughts back to love quickly and with more ease.

If I can move from such intense self-hatred to this depth of love, anyone can. I will share one tool that really helped me. I call it "The Five A's to Change."

Awareness

The first step is awareness. We can't change what we can't see. The moment we become aware of something, change has already begun. The more we practise present-moment awareness, the better we see the truth about what is helping and what is harming, whether that be our thoughts and beliefs, our unfelt emotions, judgments, projections, or physical symptoms. The best question to ask is "What is happening now?" This opens our mind to be curious about what is happening in this moment. Be open to becoming aware of your thoughts, beliefs, feelings, physical symptoms, triggers, anything at all. Be open to explore anything that you become aware of.

Acceptance

This is the main step most people miss. Instead of accepting their negative thoughts and beliefs or accepting how they feel, they pass judgment on them. We may judge ourselves or project our judgments onto someone else. Projection is a clever tactic of our ego mind. I share more about projection on Day 5 in "What We Can't See, We Can't Change." Accepting "what is" allows us to move from judging to being curious. Acceptance softens and opens our mind to another perspective. It doesn't mean we have to like what is, we just need to accept it. If we resist what is, we are holding on tightly with judgment and fear. I am sure you have heard the saying "what we resist persists." When we practise acceptance, we soften the resistance in our mind. This allows us to take ownership for how we feel or for what is happening in our life. It is okay to feel what we are feeling and at the same time be willing and open to feel differently. When we accept "what is," we become open to change. Here are some examples of ways to practise acceptance: "It is what it is and it is okay." "I am where I am and it is okay." "I am feeling anger and it is okay." "I am feeling sad and it is okay."

Allowance

Another step most people will skip, which only leads to frustration or self-doubt, is allowance. Give yourself permission to feel how you feel about what is happening. Remember that your thoughts and beliefs have been programmed and operating most of your life. Allow the thoughts to rise up and imagine you could for-give them for healing. The process of for-giving allows us to set an intention to let go and offer over our thoughts in exchange for another perspective. Make space to feel your emotions so that they can rise up and out. Emotions are meant to be felt not held or stuffed down inside. Feel your feelings to free yourself from them. Allow your thoughts to rise up into your awareness so they aren't hidden tapes playing in the background. It is our hidden thoughts and beliefs that create most of our pain. Practising awareness and allowance is like running a virus scan on a computer. Once you know there is a virus (a negative thought), you can run a program to remove it. Unfelt feelings are also like viruses causing us to react to life instead of respond to it. Allow space for your thoughts to be explored and your feelings to be felt so they can be cleared and healed.

Action

Action is the step most people jump to when they become aware of something they want to change. They go from awareness to taking action to change what they become aware of. The challenge is that, if they skip acceptance and allowance, most times the action they take to change something is not sustainable. The other aspect to consider is whether the action we take comes from our head or our heart. When we follow the directions of our heart, our gut instinct, or our intuition, we will feel a deeper commitment to the action. It becomes inspired action, instead of forced reaction. Intentionally aligning our mind with our heart, our gut instinct, or our intuition becomes a powerful recipe for change. The key is to quiet the mind and listen for the inspired action that comes from the heart. This means we follow the directions of the heart as well as its timing. This is what I refer to as inspired action.

Appreciation

Practising gratitude and appreciation is great, especially when it comes to change. Gratitude opens our mind and allows us to see what is working and what is right instead of what is wrong. When we practise seeing what is going right by focusing on what we appreciate, it helps reprogram our mind for more gratitude. We can be grateful for the awareness related to the process of change or we can have appreciation for something we are learning or for something or someone we love. It is great when it is related to the current process but not necessary. Remember: focusing on just the words of gratitude and appreciation is not enough to shift your mindset. When you practise appreciation, invite the feeling of gratitude to warm your heart.

Day 4

The Judge, the Jury, and the Judgment

Day 4 ~
The Judge, the Jury, and the Judgment

What if I said everything we do, feel, or say stems from judgment? Do you judge others? Do you judge yourself? Even if you didn't answer yes for one or both of those last two questions, you could be judging yourself as guilty or innocent, good or bad, right or wrong.

What if I said all judgment comes from the same source? It comes from our programmed mind, also known as our ego mind.

In every moment we are either observing or judging. As Day 3 "Born Innocent, Programmed Guilty" explains, we are born to observe; we are programmed to judge.

Right now your programmed mind is judging what I am saying as right or wrong, true or false, or your mind is totally distracted and squirming to change your focus to something else. Perhaps your mind is beginning to wander onto any topic other than this one. I will give you fair warning. I am about to poke the sleeping bear.

Fear of judgment from themselves and from others is a huge block for most people. It will keep some playing small, afraid to shine brightly in this world. For others, their fear of judgment will be their driving motivation to prove to others they can do it, they are worthy, or that they can overcome all obstacles.

I have done a lot of work around releasing judgment and consciously shifting my mindset around how I look upon the world. When I am with a client, I have no judgment. I have no judging thoughts because I am in alignment with my heart. I am deeply observing the energy, emotions, images, visions, and sensations while tuning into my client. Judgment does not exist. I hold a sacred space as I am shown their root blocks.

I am an intuitive healer. As you read those words, chances are you are passing judgment in your mind. Passing judgment is a habit of our programmed mind that I am about to challenge. I can see dis-ease in another person's body. I can feel others' emotions and physical pain in my body as if they were my own. I can sense the layers beneath and behind everything they are saying and feeling. Some would call me a modern day witch. Back in the day, I would have been burned at the stake for my gift, because others couldn't understand it; but more accurately, they were terrified because they judged it as unsafe, wrong, evil, or unnatural.

I can sense others' judgments of me and of the world when I tune in and I can see what is behind the judging thoughts. On some level, we believe judging others keeps us feeling safe and protected, but the truth is judging others keeps us imprisoned by fear. This often paralyzes us.

~

Judging others keeps us imprisoned by paralyzing fear.

~

I lived in fear most of my life. I was terrified to be myself and to let others see or know my real self. I had a power inside that kept me running and hiding. I ran from my gift, denied it, hid it for most of my life, first because I judged it myself.

Because I didn't understand it, I thought I was being punished. I believed I was cursed. And second because I was terrified about what others would think, say, or do if they found out.

How many times have you let your fear of judgment stop you? I bet you can't even begin to count. How many times has the fear of judgment motivated you? "I'll show them."

The good news is we can't feel judged if we don't fear judgment. Judgment is at the root of all our fears. Without judgment, we would not be afraid of anything. We would simply be present, observing the world in front of us.

~

Without judgment, we would not be afraid of anything.

~

We are born naturally observant before our minds are programmed to judge. We judge everything. Our mind is also programmed to fear judgment. So how do we stop judgment? We begin within our own mind.

Most people focus energy on their fear of judgment instead of on their own thoughts of judgment. If everyone in the world focused on stopping their own thoughts of judgment, the world would no longer be judgmental. If we each changed our own mind's programming instead of worrying about what others are judging, we would make the most progress in the shortest amount of time.

Let me break it down a bit. Judgment without a pre-conceived story or personal opinion is simply an observation. In order to observe the world without judgment, we need to look at everything as if we know nothing. The problem is that we think we know what we don't know. Our mind thinks it knows, but we only know what we were taught to know. The mind gathers knowledge and that knowledge can be true or false. How do we know if the knowledge we hold is true? We can't really. It is all based on our opinions and beliefs. Where did our opinions and beliefs come from? We were taught how to perceive and what to believe through our programming.

Our mind thinks it knows, but our heart knows. Our heart has no judgment because our heart has no thoughts, beliefs, or stories about anything. It allows us to be deeply present without history. When we filter everything we see through the lens of our heart, we can observe, be fully present, and be mindful. With quiet stillness in our mind, our heart can observe the world without judgment.

One of my mentors and motivational speaker Les Brown says, "When your desires and your beliefs are not in alignment, you will always manifest what you believe."

~

If we simply let our mind take the passenger seat and allow our heart to drive and lead, our experience of life would instantly change.

~

The challenge is we were programmed to live and lead with our logical mind, to think things through, to weigh the pros and cons, and to analyze every decision. If we simply let our mind take the passenger seat and allow our heart to drive and lead, our experience of life would instantly change. If we choose to see the world through our heart's eye—our insight—we are able to observe without judgment.

Try it for a few minutes. Look around the room and find something to look at that you feel somewhat neutral about. At first you will still have some level of judgment occurring in your mind because it is such a habit. Do your best to simply observe an object (a chair, for example) and invite the mind to be quiet. It might help to say, "I have placed the meaning I have on this chair. I think I know about this chair but what if I don't really know anything about this chair?"

Now imagine bringing your awareness down into your heart and looking through the lens of observation. Allow curiosity to soften and open your mind. You may begin to notice other details about the chair that you hadn't noticed before. You may still find some judgments coming in. Place those thoughts aside and see if you can observe the object as if you were looking at it for the first time. This is an easier practice when your focus is on something you feel neutral about. Once you practise, you can start to change your point of focus to other things you are more attached to or that you have some opinions about. It will take some practice to re-program your mind but the peace of mind it will create will be well worth the effort. It will also foster more open, vulnerable, and authentic connections with others.

Remember that we think we know what we don't know. This thinking closes our minds and our hearts. If we try on and embrace the idea that we have no flippin' clue about anything, we can open our minds and be willing to see the world differently. That also includes being able to see ourselves differently. When we observe without judgment, we can see others and observe life through a lens of love and compassion. When we make a conscious choice to stop judging ourselves and stop judging others, we stop judgment right at the source—our own minds. Imagine if we all did that all together, all at once; all judgment would cease instantly.

Day 5

What We Can't See, We Can't Change

Day 5 ~
What We Can't See, We Can't Change

We can't change what we can't see and most people don't want to see what they most need to change. I often say I help others see the invisible. I help my clients see what is in their blind spots. I shine light on the dark corners of their mind and bring into their awareness what they need to see so that they can change the behaviours that are not serving them in order to heal.

Let me begin by explaining resistance. I define resistance as the gap between what our mind thinks and what our heart knows. When the mind and heart are in alignment—in sync—there is no gap; therefore, no resistance. When our mind thinks it knows (in other words, it holds a belief) and it is not in alignment with the knowing in our heart, there is a gap; hence there will be resistance. The bigger the gap, the bigger the expression of resistance will be.

Resistance can show up as procrastination, avoidance, heaviness, depression, fear, anger, resentment, frustration, boredom, doors being closed, a busy signal on a phone call, computers crashing, blame, guilt, feeling blah, sadness; the list goes on and on. Essentially, resistance is a feeling that something is off or not going the way we planned or intended. Resistance is not wrong or bad; it is simply an invitation to pause and reflect. In other words, resistance is our friend pointing us to what we need to see in order to align with what we know in our heart.

~

Resistance is our friend pointing us to what we need to see in order to align with what we know in our heart. When we resist something, we will use projection as the mechanism to avoid the thing we are resisting.

~

When we are afraid to look within or we are really attached to our thoughts and beliefs, we are resisting. When we resist something, we will use projection as the mechanism to avoid the thing we are resisting.

We use projection when we don't want to face something within ourselves. We project or cast blame out onto others or out into the world so we feel better. The challenge is that projection offers only temporary relief as a Band-Aid on the wound that never heals. When we project and cast blame outwardly, we are avoiding taking ownership for our own stuff, which leads to guilt and feeling bad again so we project once more. It is a self-defeating cycle of projection that leaves us running on a hamster wheel and keeps us separate from everyone.

Bear with me on this one. You may feel detached, uninterested, and highly resistant to this piece. When I first heard about projection it was difficult to wrap my head around it, probably because I had such strong resistance to taking a good honest look at how I used projection in my own life.

In a nutshell, here is how it works.

We feel bad and we want to feel better, so we judge and project blame onto someone or something. We feel better temporarily, until guilt sinks in, then we feel bad again. When we feel bad we want to feel better, so we judge and resist and project and the self-defeating cycle continues.

As long as our own stuff is projected outward onto someone else, we can't see it so we can't heal it. Our ego mind will project what it doesn't want us to see and heal. As long as it is over there, it is out of our reach to heal and remains in our blind spot.

Let me give you an example of projection from my life to help paint the picture. I had been in a long-term relationship for about five years when things started to get difficult. We were growing apart and we had different interests. I was unhappy in our relationship, but I wasn't willing to let it go. When I look back, I can clearly see the pattern of self-sabotage that played out in that relationship. Essentially, I would make it so hard for my boyfriend to be with me that I was sure he would want to leave, he would break up with me, I could blame him for leaving, and I would be the victim.

Let me explain it in terms of the projection cycle.

I would feel bad because I wasn't happy in the relationship anymore and I felt it was meant to end. I resisted that because I didn't want to be the one to do the breaking up. I didn't want to look like the bad guy. At that point in my life I was used to playing the victim.

I would project and blame him for not spending enough time with me or not paying enough attention to me or spending money on alcohol and cigarettes.

I would feel better temporarily because I cast the blame on him.

Then I would feel guilty and try to make up for it by being nice, cooking him dinner, or buying him beer. That usually backfired because it was coming from a place of fear not love. I would feel bad, because I still had underlying guilt, which was really my resistance to facing the fact that the relationship was meant to end but I didn't want to be the one to end it.

Then I would project blame again and convince myself that it was his fault. If only he would change then the relationship would be good and I would feel better. And the cycle would continue over and over again, with me subconsciously hoping that finally he would break up with me and I would feel like a victim, which of course only led to another projection cycle.

After our eventual breakup, I recognized this victim mentality within myself and was able to write a letter and take full ownership for my part in the relationship's demise. I shifted from being a victim of life to feeling empowered by life. I was willing to feel all my past hurt and trauma, and heal the self-destructive patterns around that relationship and others.

I saw clearly that I was choosing partners who, I thought, needed me to save them. For the longest time, I was attracted to guys who either abused alcohol or drugs, were mostly unemployed, or those I thought needed me to help them heal their past hurts. The choices all stemmed from my feelings of abandonment around my dad's absence when I was young. I wanted to rescue them and be the hero so I could feel better about myself. I couldn't save my dad, but I could try and save them. Of course that never worked. I always ended up hurting them and myself more in the end.

When I finally created awareness and broke this pattern, I met my husband. He is a gentle, kind, loving, supportive partner and such an incredible gift in my life. When I changed my perspective, let go of being the victim, and opened my heart to another way to be in relationship, I saw him, I really saw him and the rest is history.

So we can begin to see how the projection, blame, and guilt cycle can keep us looping in repetitive self-destructive patterns in our life. We need two things to break the cycle of projection. The first is awareness and the second is willingness mixed with some courage. If we don't practise awareness and we aren't willing to see our part in the pattern, we will be stuck on the hamster wheel of projection forever. The moment we become aware, even just by being introduced to this cycle, change has already begun, and the resulting courageous willingness can carry us through to a full circle of healing.

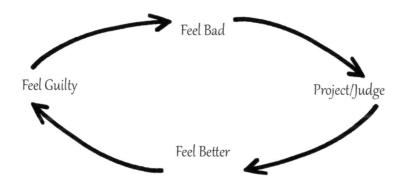

I spoke about awareness when I introduced the Five A's of Change on Day 3 "Born Innocent, Programmed Guilty." It would be worth reading or reviewing that tool again as it can lead to faster results in unwinding from this cycle. You can have awareness at any point within the cycle to break the repetitive pattern.

You can become aware of when you are feeling bad.

You may become aware of casting blame on someone or something else.

You may become aware of feeling bad and suddenly feeling better when you cast blame.

You may become aware of feeling guilty.

Anywhere in the cycle, there is the potential to create

awareness and stop the cycle. Once you have awareness ask yourself:

What am I trying to avoid feeling?

What are my judging thoughts?

What thoughts of blame are playing out in my head?

The work it takes to break these cycles is so worth it. The miracles and freedom that result are life changing. Soften your mind and open your heart so you can be free to love and be loved. You deserve a life you love.

Day 6

Mirrors Can Either Free Us or Feed Our Judgments

Day 6 ~
Mirrors Can Either Free Us or Feed Our Judgments

I can speak about two kinds of mirrors when it comes to judgments: the mirrors we look into every morning and the mirrors that occur when we see a part of ourselves in others. Both mirrors can be used intentionally to free us from judgments.

Let's begin with the actual mirror in the bathroom. When you look in the bathroom mirror, what do you see? What are the first thoughts that come into your mind? Do you look at what is right or do you judge what is wrong?

Most people use mirrors to feed their self-judgment. They pick themselves apart for every blemish, every hair out of place, the size and shape of their body parts, and how they look compared to others. This is learned behaviour and programming. As young children, we didn't use mirrors for knocking ourselves down. Instead, we were fascinated to see our own reflection mirroring our every move and expression.

I am sure some of you have seen the little girl with blonde curly hair named Jessica on YouTube doing positive affirmations in the mirror. A clip of her video was used in a Maxwell House commercial. As she looks at herself in the mirror, Jessica enthusiastically proclaims all that she likes in her life. It is inspiring and at the same time quite the opposite of how most people greet themself in the mirror.

Growing up my own self-talk was full of extreme judgment and hatred toward myself. I suffered with anorexia and bulimia for years and every time *I* looked in the mirror, it was like looking at a funhouse mirror with the distorted image. Even though I was only ninety-two pounds soaking wet, I still saw a young girl who needed to lose more weight. I based my distorted perspective on all my self-judgment and my desire to be anyone else but me. My self-hatred was extreme and deeply painful.

My relationship with mirrors has changed dramatically over the years. I began to pay attention to the thoughts that arose when I looked in the mirror. I started to see the judging thoughts as friends who were pointing to where I still needed to unwind and heal my mind. I would for-give the thoughts as I realized I had the power to choose another way of seeing myself in the mirror. It has become easier and the judgments are few and far between. At times when I am feeling low energy or when life bumps up against my leftovers, I still need to make a conscious effort to break the habit of picking myself apart in front of the mirror.

Sometimes, I look in the mirror and say, "I commit to love you, no matter what happens today." I also love using my adaptation of a quote by Macrina Wiederkehr: "I am willing to see the truth about myself, no matter how beautiful it is." I look deeply into my own eyes with the intention of connecting to my true self. I feel a sense of wholeness and oneness with my soul, heart, mind, and body. It has been a challenging process, but it works. I know if I can make the shift and change my habitual judgments, anyone can.

~

I look deeply into my own eyes with the intention of connecting to my true self. I feel a sense of wholeness and oneness with my soul, heart, mind, and body.

~

What if, the next time you find yourself in front of a mirror, you started to encourage yourself, give yourself a compliment, offer a pep talk, and be your own cheerleader? How would that feel? Probably extremely uncomfortable at first, but with some practice it can become more of a positive habit.

Now, let's look at the mirrors out in the world that come in the form of people and/or situations that trigger us and cause judgment to arise in our mind.

Imagine that the world is full of mirrors reflecting back to us what we need to see, know, and feel in order to heal. Every person, interaction, situation, and experience becomes an opportunity to look within. When we project our judgments out into the world, we can't heal or change them. They are out of our reach and in our blind spot. We can't change what we can't see.

When we use our life as a classroom and keep our minds wide open, we can build awareness around our triggers and judgments. In the light of awareness we can make change happen.

In a conversation about judging and projection, my dearest friend and soul sister, Reverend Lisa Windsor, said to me, "If you can see it in them, it must be in you." Those words really landed and became an essential tool for me to start bringing my own judgments back into my awareness to shift them. When I had a judgment about someone I would turn it around and mirror it back onto myself. Let me share an example.

I just woke up from a dream in which I was visiting the veterinary clinic where I used to work as a Veterinary Technician and Hospital Manager. I was in the kennel area and I noticed the back door wasn't closing properly. Someone had jammed some cardboard pieces into the bottom so it wouldn't lock properly. I started talking to everyone in the neighbourhood to figure out who had done this. I knew their plan was to come back after the clinic closed and steal what they wanted. I could feel anger rising up in me and I was determined to catch the person responsible. I felt very protective of my friends who owned the clinic.

Still dreaming, I finally figured out who it was, so I started searching for that individual. When I went back to the clinic to tell everyone to watch out for him, I found him in the back checking out the door and noticing it was no longer rigged to stay open. I confronted him. He had already started collecting some things to steal. I was angry and I slapped him in the face. "How dare you? Why can't you just make an honest living like everyone else? Why do you have to steal?" I was trying to get the attention of the other staff but no one could hear me, so I threw him into one of the dog cages. I felt disgust, resentment, and anger. He deserved to be punished but I knew that because he hadn't actually broken in he wouldn't be charged and he would get away with his potential crime.

I woke up feeling angry, annoyed, and resentful. I stayed with these feelings for a while, but they wouldn't budge. While I felt the emotional discord in my own body, I had projected it out onto the alleged crook in my dream. I started to journal about how I was feeling.

I started by listing the judgments I had toward him.

I judged him for not making an honest living.

I judged him for stealing from others.

I judged him as guilty and needing to be punished.

Then I practised the mirror technique. If I could see it in him, it must be in me. I turned all my judgments back onto myself.

I judge myself for not making an honest living.

I judge myself for stealing from others.

I judge myself as guilty and needing to be punished.

I felt a wave of guilt rise up. At first, my mind pointed the guilt outward and I felt bad for slapping him. Where was my compassion? I could see I was projecting again to avoid what I was really feeling, so I turned the guilt back onto myself once more and looked a little more deeply.

Suddenly I had a memory of stealing from a store when I was young. I started stealing candy with a friend from the local convenience store. No one caught us. When we got away with it a few more times, I started trying to steal bigger things. It didn't take long before I was caught for stealing. I felt so guilty and a deep shame filled my heart.

The clerk made me call my mom to tell her what I had done, but I just stayed quiet when she answered. I couldn't bring myself to speak the words. The guilt and shame were eating me up inside. I felt so heavy because I would disappoint my mom. I had tried so hard to uphold the image of being the good little girl. That image came crashing down as the guilty verdict came flooding into my mind. My ego persona "Judge Judy" was fully awakened in my mind and was ready to kick some butt. In the end the clerk called my mom and she grounded me for two weeks. That didn't really feel like punishment enough, so my "Judge Judy" gave me a life sentence of feeling guilty: I would need to spend my lifetime making up for my crime. I continued to punish myself and lived with the guilt for decades.

Almost twenty years later, I saw the store clerk at a friend's house gathering. Immediately I felt the shame rise up again. He recognized me and tried to talk to me, but I pretended not to know him and left. I avoided feeling that awful judgment of guilty, and once again buried it deep.

Tonight as I was journaling, I could feel another layer of guilt and shame washing up for healing. It had been years since I really reflected on that experience as a child, so I brought myself back to the memory and focused on how I felt. My body tensed up even more. As I sat, feeling into my heart and solar plexus, I could feel a dense heaviness in my heart. I softened around it and invited the energy to move. As I brought the intention of for-giving myself, everything began to soften and the energy shifted. Not all of it moved but most of it shifted.

I went back to my journal and explored the leftovers. In just a few words, I knew I was meant to expose this shame-filled childhood story in this book. I can't keep it hidden any longer. Exposing it by sharing it frees me and hopefully will inspire others to for-give their past as well. In this moment, I feel a sense of relief and compassion for the little girl who learned from her mistake. The last layer has been released, all thanks to a dream that I was willing to use as a mirror for my own healing.

The mirror exercise is a powerful tool to shift our habit of judging others and use it to heal ourselves . When we take ownership of our judgments and are willing to look within and clear our own leftovers, we free ourselves and, at the same time, we open our hearts to see others through a lens of love and compassion.

So the next time you have a judgment about someone else, turn it back onto yourself. If you see it in them, it must be in you.

If your judgment is "They are such a bully," ask yourself, "How am I a bully?"

You may be surprised by what you uncover. It may not be easy to take an honest look within, but I promise you it will be well worth it.

Day 7

Is There a Healthy Expression of Anger?

Day 7 ~
Is There a Healthy Expression of Anger?

We learn how to hate just the same way we learn how to love. While love is our natural state, our environment and external programming determine how we deal with our negative emotions as well as our capacity to love.

Nelson Mandela said, "No one is born hating another person because of the color of his skin, or his background, or his religion. People must learn to hate, and if they can learn to hate, they can be taught to love, for love comes more naturally to the human heart than its opposite."

Anger, resentment, rage, and hatred are blocks to love. Negative emotions come with a lot of judgment or a fear of judgment. Many people do not know how to process these heavy negative emotions. Even those who have fits of rage and outwardly express hate are doing so because that is part of their learned programming, but also because they don't know how to process their own negative emotions in a healthy way.

These heavy emotions are becoming harder to hide, contain within, and keep at bay. It is as though a bubbling volcano is ready to erupt. In fact, many people process anger that way. Unexpressed anger becomes a cesspool of resentment, which eventually becomes a bout of rage. Eventually the volcano needs to erupt. When something happens in our environment that bumps up against our accumulated boiling cesspool of unexpressed feelings, it causes us to blow up. Instead of feeling our own unexpressed feelings, we project them out into the world and cast our anger out as words and/or violence.

Before I explain how we can process this long-held accumulation of negative emotions, I would like to explain the idea of healthy and unhealthy expressions of anger. When I was a child, I was taught that anger was bad—to be angry was to be violent. While I never experienced any physical violence in my own home, I grew to believe that anger equalled violence. My interpretation of that falsehood was that anger was unacceptable and shouldn't be outwardly expressed. I learned to hold it in and bury it deep inside. I learned to bite my tongue and swallow that bitter pill of resentment.

It wasn't until I was a student in an experiential counselling program that I learned there were healthy and unhealthy expressions of anger. At first, I was baffled by this idea. It boggled my mind. It was like someone telling me the sky was purple and not blue as I had thought. Then I felt a huge relief as though the world had just been lifted off my shoulder. I could finally learn how to release years of built-up resentment and rage in a healthy way. Mostly, I had directed my rage and hatred toward myself. Self-blame, self-punishment, and self-destructive behaviours were my coping mechanisms. In that moment of realization while sitting in the counselling program, I had hope that one day I would be free of it. I was determined to release every last bit of anger and resentment. It was interfering with my ability to love and receive love.

So what does a healthy expression of anger look like? This is a question I tried on for years personally as well as exploring it with my clients. I have learned that even if we give ourselves permission to express our anger verbally in the moment that the energy of anger can be processed in as little as fifteen seconds. Something as simple as saying, "I am feeling angry because ..." is sometimes enough to clear it from our mind and body. It is important to just let the thoughts rise up and out as words without censoring them and feel the emotions behind the words. When we do this, the words we say to ourselves are meant to feel emotionally charged; that is how we free ourself from the anger and upset behind them. Here are some examples of this exercise; you can do it on your own.

"I feel angry because no one seems to care about my needs and everyone is so selfish."

"I feel angry because my parents never loved me the way I wanted them to."

"I feel angry because my boyfriend is cheating on me."

"I feel angry because my life is falling apart."

"I feel angry because no one listens to me."

Owning how we feel is empowering. There will be times when we also need to voice our upset or anger to others, which means finding the courage to have those sweaty-palm conversations with the individual directly. Alternatively, it could mean talking about how you feel with a trustworthy friend who can hold space for you to express yourself.

~

Owning how we feel is empowering.

~

One of the most effective tools I offer my clients to move anger and dense long-held emotions, thoughts, and beliefs is an "expression session." This is where I hold space for them to bring all their hidden thoughts and beliefs into the light for healing. They get to share, express, say, yell, scream, growl, swear, and cry; they say whatever they need to say in order to release what they are holding inside. There is no conversation, just a nonjudgmental space for expression. If the anger is directed at a specific person or situation, I encourage my client to use the language that makes it sound like they are speaking directly to that individual.

This type of session is extremely cathartic as all the unspoken thoughts and feelings that have been plaguing a person come to the surface and are released. It works well for expressing all of our internal critical thoughts as well. Sharing our negative critical self-talk out loud exposes it and releases it. I often say it is like throwing it all up. I encourage clients to keep going until they feel as though they have emptied it all out, to the point where there is nothing left to say. Most of the time, there is an underlying fear, grief, or a sense of loss hidden beneath the anger. An expression session is a powerful tool that requires a compassionate witness who can be fully present, nonjudgmental, and who won't get caught up in the words and the story. If you need support in releasing anger or other pent-up feelings, contact me for an expression session.

Another way to release what is bottled up inside you is to write an eff-you letter. It is a letter to the individual that is NOT to be sent. This is for your eyes only. Let it all out and say what you have always wanted to say or need to say. Once you feel you have emptied out all the words onto paper, burn the copy or delete it. I cannot stress this enough—it is for your eyes only! When you burn the letter or delete it, set an intention to let it all go. It may be helpful to follow up your eff-you letter with a forgiveness letter.

Day 8

When Life Bumps Up Against Your Leftovers

Day 8 ~
When Life Bumps Up Against Your Leftovers

Our life is a classroom designed for our healing and for waking each of us up to be a full expression of our true Self. It is designed to trigger us, jolt us, pinch us, knock us down, empower us, and propel us into inspired action. Life is happening for us.

Life is a gift that brings up to the surface all of our leftover unresolved issues, resentments, emotions, and traumas so we can look at them and heal them fully and completely. It is also designed for us to remember the truth of who we are. All of the triggers and upsets are simply blocks to love. When we process those bumps in the road we learn how to love deeply once again. The key is to embrace each one and process and heal all of them, leaving no stone unturned.

~

The key is to embrace, process, and heal all of our leftover unresolved issues, resentments, emotions, and traumas, leaving no stone unturned.

~

Last night I watched a movie on Netflix called *To the Bone*. It was a story about a twenty-year-old girl with anorexia. As I watched the movie, I felt a deep connection to her daily struggles in obsessing about food and fighting her internal demons. My heart sank when everyone around her kept telling her to just eat, thinking that was the issue. Every time I heard someone say something about food, I heard myself say, "It's not about food." The internal workings of an eating disorder are complicated and even though food is the point of focus, it is not the root issue.

As the movie continued, I was reminded of the internal workings of my own battle with anorexia and bulimia in my late teens and early twenties. I could relate so much to the story and I felt a deep empathy when the girl spiralled down in weight so much that she was close to dying.

During one scene at the very end, tears starting pouring out of my eyes as though a faucet had been turned on. I started bawling and sobbing uncontrollably. Yes, I was crying about the movie, but I was crying about all my leftovers. I felt a raw vulnerability and a deep surrender as a layer of grief, loss, and defeat washed up through me. I remember my lowest point, physically and emotionally. I remember when I hit rock bottom and my eating disorder spiralled out of my control. I remember curling up in a ball on the floor and praying for something, someone to reach out their hand and help me out of the dark hole I had buried myself in. I had been yearning for someone to pick me up and rock me gently and tell me I was going to be okay.

As I am writing this, more tears are flowing. I am reminded of the image I was upholding during that time. I was a Registered Veterinary Technician who had graduated with honours and received several awards. I was a part-time fitness instructor teaching others how to be healthy and fit, and my biggest secret—something I hid for years and was convinced I had control over—was suddenly taking over my entire life. The most painful thing for me was my fear that I couldn't keep it hidden and secret. It was as though I was living a double life, pretending to be one way, yet living in an internal hell at the same time.

When I woke up this morning, I pulled some angel cards. I received the words "authenticity, strength, and transformation." As I tuned in for messages around these cards, I saw myself writing about my experience of watching the movie. I hesitated and resisted for a moment. Then I heard the words "raw authenticity is transformational." So I gathered my strength and courage and began this chapter.

As I continue to create space for the leftover tears, loss, grief, heaviness, judgment, and fear to wash up, I feel deeply vulnerable. In one way it feels like a lifetime ago; on the other hand, in this moment it is real, raw, and fresh. So I allow space to feel that as well. I am willing to feel it all to heal it all. I don't want to carry any of it anymore. So I will continue to allow the emotions to express themselves, and the feelings to be felt and the judgments to wash up and out of the deep recesses of my mind until there is nothing left. I will leave no stone unturned.

~

I am willing to feel it all to heal it all.

~

When life bumps up against our leftovers, let it. Embrace it. It is an opportunity and a gift in disguise. It requires our courage to face it and to ask for help, our willingness to feel it, and our strength to surrender so we can let it go.

So the next time you feel triggered, stop and take a breath, look within and ask yourself, "What am I really feeling underneath this trigger?" Be willing to look deeper than at the obvious feeling at the surface layer.

Ask yourself, "What leftover is trying to rise up inside me for healing?" Look at the thoughts and memories that are rising up with it. They will point to what you are meant to heal. Then create some space for the expression and release all of it. Freedom is just on the other side of feeling.

When we use our life as our classroom, we can embrace all of life's experiences with intention to awaken our greatest expression of self. We will feel a deep sense of purpose and find meaning in every moment of every day.

When we clear all our own leftovers and our obstacles to love, we can be the compassionate witness for others. We can hold them tenderly and authentically in their most vulnerable moments, and we can reassure them they are going to be okay. We can express true compassion and empathy for others and that is a recipe that will unite us in love for each other.

Day 9

Asking for Help Is an Act of Courage

Day 9 ~
Asking for Help Is an Act of Courage

It requires more courage to ask for help than it does to "go it alone." Society teaches us that we should be strong and independent and we should persevere. It also teaches us that showing any sign of weakness is detrimental and the worst possible thing we can do. We are taught that asking for help is a sign of weakness, where in truth it is the opposite: it is an act of courage.

I grew up believing I had to be independent, to have all the answers and appear as though I had my life together. While I definitely upheld that image on the outside the best I could, my inside world was full of fear, negative self-talk thoughts, and a lot of pain and suffering. I isolated myself and convinced myself that no one would understand or care about how I was feeling. My own self-judgment was extreme and it caused a lot of my own suffering. I felt as though I just had to suck it up and figure things out myself. All the while that I yearned for deep connection, love, and nurturing attention, I was also terrified of it.

Many people judge asking for help as a sign of vulnerability and weakness. The opposite is actually true. My mentor and motivational speaker Les Brown always told me, "Ask for help. Not because you are weak but because you want to remain strong." Vulnerability is a sign of strength and asking for help shows true courage. We are not meant to do this all alone. It is our tendency to isolate ourselves that creates our deepest pain and continued suffering. Not asking for help isolates and separates us from others. Asking for help connects us.

~

It is our tendency to isolate ourselves that creates our deepest pain and continued suffering. Not asking for help isolates and separates us from others. Asking for help connects us.

~

Asking for help is a gift. It not only empowers us, it is an opportunity for others to extend love. Most people love helping others. It is also a gift to fully receive what is given. Imagine giving someone a gift and they place it on the table and refuse to open it. How would that feel? Every time you are not willing to receive you are placing their gift on the table and refusing to open it.

I have a fresh story to share that relates exactly to this concept. About a month ago, I received an email from a yoga instructor asking if I offer any discounts on my Fertility Yoga Teacher Training online course. I tuned into my heart and felt a clear yes to offer her a $100 discount. I had the thought "what a generous gift" and sent her an email with the news. She met it with gratitude and accepted my offer. I emailed her a PayPal invoice with the discounted price.

A month passed and I remembered that she hadn't paid the invoice to register. As I was writing this chapter, I took a break and checked my email, because I had sent her a reminder email about the invoice just the day before, asking her to let me know either way so I could cancel the invoice if she is no longer interested. Part of me expected she had forgotten and just needed a reminder. When I received her email saying she would like to cancel for now, I was surprised.

The very first thought I heard in my mind was, "What? You are not going to take advantage of the discount?" That thought was quickly followed by, "Well, I won't be offering the discount again. This was her only chance so she missed out." I could feel some tension building in the centre of my chest and my ego mind was ready to pounce and take me into a wormhole of judgment. I knew I had a choice to either let my thoughts continue or to place my attention inward and feel the emotions beneath those thoughts.

As I tuned into my chest, I felt a wave of disappointment followed by a heavy sadness in my heart. I had extended a gift and she had refused to open it. She wasn't willing to receive it. The heaviness grew as I felt the density of all the times I have extended a gift that wasn't received or wasn't received in the way I intended. For many years, I had spent time and energy on helping others who weren't willing to help themselves—all those people I had wanted to help but couldn't. I continue to have tears as I am typing. The grief continues to wash up and out.

All along I thought I was giving her a gift but it turns out she was actually extending a gift to me. Without this interaction, I wouldn't have looked within and felt the collection of past hurt and grief from the gifts I have extended that were never received. I wanted to save the world as a child so there were many. Then suddenly, I felt a wave of grief from all the gifts that I myself have refused to open and receive with my whole heart. All my unopened gifts, the gifts I denied myself because I felt unworthy and undeserving.

Curiously, I didn't feel guided to respond to her email, but I did send a blessing from my heart to hers. I was willing to receive her gift: the gift of healing, the gift of awareness, the gift of surrender, and the gift of non-attachment. This one email exchange was full of so much potential and I was willing to open it fully and receive it all.

I knew it took courage for her to initially ask for help in the way of a discount, but I have come to recognize that it takes just as much courage, if not more, to receive the help when it is extended. Whether it is in response to us asking for help or someone offering their help out of the blue, it takes courage to say yes and be open to receive. We may be able to conjure up the courage to finally ask for help, but if we aren't open to receive it when it arrives, it remains an unopened gift.

The real joy and pleasure in giving comes from knowing the gift you are extending is being received. I often say giving is receiving, and receiving is giving. There is no difference, because when you give you receive and when you receive you give. There is always an exchange going both ways. Even when you give a gift anonymously, you receive the gift of knowing you made a difference in someone else's life. Even when the gift is not received and opened, there is still a gift you can receive. As I share in this story, the gift we receive back can often be disguised as an opportunity to heal our leftovers and our past hurts.

Asking for help is an act of courage and so is being open to receive. For many, giving comes at a sacrifice to self, because there is an imbalance between giving to others and giving to self. Many of us find it easy to give but much harder to receive. We often judge ourselves unworthy, undeserving and/or not important; we are programmed to believe that receiving is being selfish.

For most people, our hearts are wide open to give but closed to receiving. How do we change that? We pay attention to the conversation in our heads so that we can challenge our programmed thoughts and the judgments that rise up. We can make a choice to be more open to receiving throughout the day. If someone compliments you, soften your heart and say "thank you." If someone holds a door open for you, receive the gift of a kind gesture with a simple "thank you." Don't just say the words, feel the gratitude in your heart and let it warm you from the inside. If someone smiles at you, let it land in your heart as you smile back. If someone gives you a hug, hug them back with a soft open heart. It sounds easy, but it will not be easy in the beginning. As you practise, it will become more familiar and eventually more natural.

We are each worthy of love. We each deserve to receive the gifts that life holds for us. We each matter. Every one of us plays an essential role in this world. Yes, every single one of us. We each have a unique gift in our heart to extend. When we open our hearts to receive, we are giving a gift to all of humanity.

Maya Angelou wrote, "You can't give from an empty cup." I like to teach "We can't give from an empty heart." One of the principles I teach in my book *Heart Led Living ~ When Hard Work Becomes Heart Work* is "Fill Your Heart First."

When we ask for help, we have a choice to open our hearts to receive love from others. It is a choice to fill our heart. The key is to fill our heart enough that we can give from the overflow and never experience the feeling of depletion or self-sacrifice. We are no help to anyone when we feel empty and depleted. Asking for help allows us to sustain our own energy and at the same time creates a connection with others.

Yes, it takes courage. Yes, it may feel unnatural but only at first. I assure you it is the most natural thing once you get past the old programming in your mind. Go ahead—ask for help.

All it takes is twenty seconds of courage. Take a deep breath, gather your courage, and take the leap.

Day 10

What Image Are You Upholding?

Day 10 ~
What Image Are You Upholding?

The image we uphold in this world is a hidden self-judgment that leads to the main source of our pain and suffering.

Who am I?

Who are you?

Who do you pretend to be?

Who do you want to be?

Who are you when no one is watching?

I find it so curious that most people spend energy trying to be someone other than who they are. Many of us are programmed to believe we were born to be someone else, other than who we are. We are each born as our unique self, yet we spend a lifetime resisting that. Why? So we can fit in? So we can feel like we belong? We are not meant to fit in. We are meant to stand out. We are each meant to be a unique expression of self.

The judgment that we are not good enough the way we are is strongly portrayed in almost every advertisement, infomercial, magazine, and movie. This programming is deeply effective in our society. We are taught that we are not good enough, strong enough, smart enough, worthy enough, skinny enough, skilled enough, pretty enough, tall enough, perfect enough; and the list goes on and on and on.

Over the years we gather evidence of what is acceptable and what is unacceptable. We collect data on what others like and don't like about us. We strive to be accepted by everyone and we yearn to feel a sense of belonging. We judge ourselves over and over again based on what others think, what articles say, and what pictures portray, all the while striving to be anyone other than who we really are. We are trying to be a better version of ourselves because our current version isn't good enough.

Our fear of judgment, and even more so of our self-judgment, drives our fear-based desire to live up to the expectations the world has placed on us. Here is the kicker: we will never ever, ever, ever live up to those expectations because it is not the world that has placed those expectations on us; we have done that to ourselves by buying into the world's unrealistic version of what it means to be ourselves. We have put that pressure on ourselves by choosing to believe everyone else's judgment and take it on as our own.

What image are you upholding?

Who are you trying to impress?

Whose expectations do you believe you are trying to meet?

I have spent most of my life wanting to be anyone else but me. At the same time, I spent a great deal of energy pretending to have it all together so that I wouldn't burden anyone else. It was a hard role to play because I had so much internal pain that I could only hold it together for periods of time before I would fall apart. This usually happened in the privacy of my own company. The pressure would become so intense I would explode in tears and grief. After the tears passed, I would get up, wipe my tears, brush myself off, and once again step into the image I felt the need to uphold.

After all, I didn't want to disappoint anyone.

I wanted everyone to like me and I would go to great lengths to make sure I was accepted. In most circles, I was likeable but not in all. Feeling unaccepted was a deep wound. Feeling left out created such an intense feeling of loneliness it was difficult to bear, but I had a role to play, an image to uphold, a world to save; I had no choice but to grin and bear it.

I have come to realize that not everyone is going to like me and I have made peace with that. In fact, I embrace it now as a gift. I often trigger people because I am a mirror for what they need to look at within themselves. There are times I will walk into a room and some people will see me and run the other way. Some will make eye contact but pretend they don't see me. As an intuitive healer and an empath, I can sense what is happening behind the scenes. I can sense people's hidden pains, fears, and emotions. That can be terrifying for some people, because I may be able to see what they are hiding behind the image they are upholding. They are afraid to be exposed by my x-ray vision. They are afraid that I will see the hidden skeletons in their closet. In some ways this is true, because I can pick up on what is hidden and playing in the background. However, unless I am working specifically with a client or a group, I do my best to mind my own business.

When I was younger and didn't understand my gift, I would pick up on messages coming at me from everyone in all directions. It was exhausting for me and not helpful for others. While I do have the ability to energetically eavesdrop or read behind the headlines, I choose to respect others' privacy and honour my gift by using it with clear intentions to tune in and help when I am meant to.

We are all mirrors for others and that will attract some people to us for healing, whereas others will lash out and project blame onto us to make themselves feel better. Some will run the other way because they are afraid to face their own wounds and leftovers. When I see someone withdraw and run away from me, I bless them. I send them love and see them as capable. I pray they find the individual who is meant to support them in seeing their shadows and facing their fears. I remember I am not meant to help everyone.

Some of the images I upheld were:

The good little girl

The helper

The healthy fitness guru

The successful business owner

The healer

I lived much of my life feeling like an imposter, pretending to be one way on the outside and feeling another way on the inside. When I first started my career as a fitness instructor I was suffering from anorexia and bulimia. I would teach others about how to eat healthy and be fit, yet I was barely eating any food and obsessively weighing myself several times a day. I felt like a fraud but I convinced myself that I was helping others so it was okay.

~

Through the imposter syndrome, we live one way, upholding an image in the world, but we feel a different way on the inside, behind the scenes when no one is looking.

~

Through the imposter syndrome, we live one way, upholding an image in the world, but we feel a different way on the inside, behind the scenes when no one is looking. We feel like a fraud and as long as we uphold an image that we can't live up to or we don't reach out for help, we will continue to feel trapped. To this day, my ego mind still continues to try and create new images to uphold, by convincing me I need to live up to the expectations of the world. Sometimes it catches me off guard and I go along for the ride until I realize what is happening and I make a choice to surrender once again. Every morning, I wake up and choose to be the most authentic version of myself. Some people will accept me and some won't and that is okay.

What are some of the images you upheld growing up?

What are some of the images you are currently upholding?

What are you protecting?

What are you afraid people will find out about you?

Are you willing to face your fears and surrender all the images you uphold so that you learn to embrace who you are meant to be?

It all begins with creating awareness and making a conscious choice to let go, surrender, and trust. There is no one else in this world that would make a better you. You are the only you that exists. The world doesn't need you to strive to be someone else. What the world needs is for you to be a full expression of YOU and nobody else but YOU.

Day 11

We are Meant to Stand Out, Not Fit In

Day 11 ~
We are Meant to Stand Out, Not Fit In

Have you ever tried to fit inside a box that was too small, contorting your limbs and squishing all your body parts just to fit in? I am sure you have seen a few entertaining videos of cats squishing themselves into small boxes or paper bags. Perhaps you made forts out of blankets and boxes when you were a child so you could tuck yourself in and hide away in your own little world. The important question to ask yourself is, "Am I still trying to fit inside the box, play small, and hide my true self from the rest of the world?"

I remember as a child building forts using furniture, pillows, and blankets. I would add my favourite stuffed animals and other comforting trinkets and I would crawl inside my own little world and feel safe for a while. While my home was safe, the rest of the world felt big, intimidating, and painful to me. As an empath and a healer, I could physically and emotionally sense and feel all the pain of others in my own body like constant thorns. I came to the conclusion that it was hard and painful to be me.

I tried to fit in and pretend to be someone other than who I was for a long time but in the end it led me on a path of more pain and suffering. Denying my unique gift as a healer was dishonouring to who I am at the core of my being. Trying to be like others instead of giving myself permission to be me created a feeling of claustrophobia that was strangling my creativity and keeping me playing small. I didn't want to stand out or make anyone feel inferior. I didn't want to outshine others, because I didn't want them to feel bad; yet at the same time I was trying to prove my worthiness and follow my dream to save the world. Growing up I wanted to save others more than I wanted to save myself. It was a constant internal tug-of-war that used up so much of my energy it was exhausting—it left me feeling helpless and disconnected from my sense of self.

It is through the lens of fear and judgment that we make decisions to go with the crowd, follow like a herd of sheep, not rock the boat, lie low, play small, be accepted, and fit in a box that doesn't stand out from the rest. We are taught to try and fit in. But, we are not meant to fit in. We are meant to stand out. If we were meant to be carbon copies of each other, we wouldn't have been born with our unique features, gifts, talents, and personalities.

~

We are taught to try and fit in. But, we are not meant to fit in. We are meant to stand out.

~

The perspective we choose and the lens we use to see life will determine what we see. Snowflakes are a great example. When we look at snow falling from the sky, we see snowflakes. From a distance, they all look the same. But when we zoom in and take a closer look, we can see that each snowflake is unique. No two snowflakes are the same. Each snowflake has unique characteristics. As a child, I was fascinated by that. Depending on your perspective, the snowflakes look the same or completely different. You can say the same thing about the leaves on a tree. When we take a closer look, each one has a uniqueness that is sometimes subtle and at other times more obvious.

Now I am not saying all of this to make us feel separate from each other, but to emphasize that we each have a unique role to play here on this Earth at this time. We are all connected at the core of who we are and at the same time we are meant to stand out and share our unique gifts with the world. As long as we are trying to be like everyone else, we will always feel inadequate and find evidence of how we are not enough. When we are trying to fit into a box that someone else built and live up to the standards that others have set, we will always fall short; we will never fit in; we will always feel like we don't belong. This creates a fundamental experience of separation.

The good news is that when we stand up, own our uniqueness by being fully authentic, we each play an essential role in the healing of the whole. Every single one of us has an essential part to play. When we watch a movie, we can see how each character adds value and depth to the overall script. If everyone were playing the same character, the movie would be a bust.

Some of us have a small role and some have a bigger role to play, but each role is essential. One person's version of playing small may be another person's version of playing big. It is not about comparing ourselves with others. Comparison is a game of judgment that makes us feel inadequate no matter what we are doing or not doing. By comparing ourselves, we will collect enough evidence to convince ourselves that we will never be, do, or have enough. Comparison always crushes creativity, insight, and intuition.

~

Comparison is a game of judgment that makes us feel inadequate no matter what we are doing or not doing; it always crushes creativity, insight, and intuition.

~

When we shift from the fear of comparison to the energy of co-operation, we shift into being a contribution to all of humanity. We honour the role each of us has to play and we are willing to contribute to the whole by playing our role fully, wholly, and completely. We return to love and harmony. We can stand strong, united in love.

Our heart holds the key and our script for our part in the play is placed inside us. So how do we get out of our head and into our heart? How do we shift our perspective and open our mind to receive the guidance from within?

It is about tuning into your heart and being truthful about how you are showing up in life.

I encourage you to ask yourself the following questions. First, take ten deep breaths. Yes, right now. Stop and take ten deep breaths. Imagine yourself in your mind knowing that you can take an elevator down into your heart. Go down, down, down deep into your heart space. As you read the following questions, let the answers come from deep within. Go with the first answer that pops into your awareness and write it down (even if it doesn't make sense).

How am I shrinking, hiding, and dimming my light?
How am I playing small?
How am I trying to fit in?
What role am I meant to play?
Am I willing to play full out?
Am I willing to play my part in the grand plan?

Am I willing to stand up and stand out and be a full authentic expression of myself?

In what areas of my life am I showing up fully to play my part?

~

I guarantee your heart knows what your part is.

~

Many of you may be wondering how to know what your part is. You can't know in your head, but I guarantee your heart knows. As long as we are using the limited programmed filters of our mind, we will never truly know how we are meant to stand out. Our mind is full of fear-based filters, judgment, and the fear of judgment, along with a long list of perceived limitations of the world.

If we drop into our heart, we can tap into a knowing that goes beyond our mind. It is a knowing that resides in our heart. It is our heart that holds the key and specific directions to our life script. All we need to do is get out of our head and into our hearts and let the directions come. As with a recipe, each ingredient will be given and each direction will be provided one step at a time.

The world doesn't need you to fit in. What the world needs is for you to play your part—stand up, stand out, and stand strong. You have a unique role and an essential part to play. The world needs you now more than ever. Are you willing to play your part?

Say YES! Just say YES!

Day 12

When We Fight to Be Right, We Will Always Feel Wrong

Day 12 ~
When We Fight to Be Right, We Will Always Feel Wrong

There is a strong emphasis placed on right and wrong in our society. It is everywhere we look. The pressure to be right and the fear of being wrong are palpable. There is so much shame attached to being wrong that we learn to fight to be right. The problem is when we fight to be right we will always feel wrong.

There are always at least two sides to every story. The two main perspectives held are right and wrong. I am right or they are right. If I am right, they are wrong. If I am wrong, they are right. We are taught discerning between right and wrong is black and white, but it is not. We can't both be right, can we? We can't both be wrong, can we? There is a grey area of interpretation, experience, programming, and intuition that influences both sides.

Now I am not interested in getting into a debate here about specific situations. My intention is simply to challenge our programmed minds to try on another perspective and explore the grey area a bit. It takes a willingness to be wrong to even begin to try on another possible perspective. So I invite you to be open and willing to be wrong, even if it is just while you are reading this. This will be uncomfortable for some people and excruciatingly painful for others. Very few if any will easily embrace this idea.

Our fight to be right is deeply rooted in our instinct to protect ourselves and others. It is like a mama grizzly bear instinct, so be gentle with yourself as we explore and unravel this concept.

There are some people who hate being wrong and, even when they know they are wrong, they fight to be right. I remember talking to a guy about Egypt and I said I have always wanted to go to Africa but that I was just not sure I would go to Egypt first. He told me, "Egypt is not in Africa." I responded, "Yes, it is." He proceeded to spend ten more minutes trying to convince me that Egypt was not in the continent of Africa and I was baffled by his stern stance. I finally took out a map. Yes, it was an old school map in an atlas, as this happened before the internet was born. I pointed to Egypt and it clearly showed its borders were in fact within the African continent.

I expected him to say, "You're right," but instead he said, "Well, that map is wrong."

I was shocked. The proof was right there in front of him, but he wasn't willing to stand down and admit he was wrong. Instead, he stood solidly in his stance of "I am right and everyone and everything else is wrong." I let it go and walked away. I knew it was a battle I couldn't win even if I was willing to take up arms and fight. I chose to agree to disagree, but silently, because I knew even if I said that, he would continue his fight to change my mind, take his side, and agree he was right.

Our fight to be right can skew our perception. We see what we want to see, which is not always actually what is happening. We can fight so hard to be right that we aren't willing to try on another perspective. We aren't willing to hear anyone else's opinion. We are right and that is that, end of story. The problem is when we fight to be right we are closed-minded and often blind to see anything else.

If our fight to be right is instinctual, then what are we

protecting? We are protecting ourselves from embarrassment, from being ridiculed and shamed. For many people, being wrong leads to punishment and can even feel like imprisonment. Being judged as wrong means we are guilty. That can lead to a life sentence, even if it is only in our minds. We condemn ourselves and strive to prove our innocence. We can turn that energy into trying to fight to be right in another area so we can try and make up for being judged wrong. It is a self-destructive cycle fed by societal pressure; it is a battle that is never ever won by either side.

~

If our fight to be right is instinctual, then what are we protecting? We are protecting ourselves from embarrassment, from being ridiculed and shamed.

~

At this point, especially on social media, it doesn't matter which side we stand for—there will be a strong opposition telling us we are wrong. So as long as we are fighting to be right, we will always feel wrong and the battle will continue. We will always feel wrong because in their eyes we are wrong, even if we are right.

I have decided to stop fighting to be right. I stopped trying to prove anything anymore, to others and more importantly to myself. I am done fighting everyone and everything. I dropped my weapons and my armour and I surrendered my need to be right. This is still a work in progress. Every once in a while, my need to be right rises up like a forceful mother bear and I have to take a deep breath and declare to myself, "I am totally willing to be wrong."

When I am totally willing to be wrong, it ends my fight to be right and it gives no further ammunition to the other person. Being willing to be wrong removes the drive from my ego mind and I soften into observation without judgment. I am defenceless and in my defencelessness I am free. Defencelessness frees my mind, heart, and soul. It creates space for me to make a conscious choice for love and I see everyone through a different lens.

~

When I am totally willing to be wrong, it ends my fight to be right and it gives no further ammunition to the other person.

~

It is no longer a lens of guilty until proven innocent. It is no longer a lens of right and wrong. It is no longer a lens of judgment. It is a lens of love and compassion. I can see someone else's fear beyond their fight to be right. I can see their driving force. And beyond all of that, I can see their innocence. I can see their call for love. They are not really fighting to be right; they are calling for love and, in my defencelessness, I can answer it fully and wholeheartedly. Sometimes, that looks like no action and I say nothing. Sometimes, that means I agree to disagree. And sometimes, I might even say, "You are right." I trust my intuition and I am willing to play my part and extend love in the way they need it at the time. I see their tender heart and meet them right there in their wound and love them. Whether they are right or wrong, I simply meet them with love. It is not about changing them or their stance, but changing the way I see them. I have witnessed some beautiful miracles in those tender moments of defencelessness, and each one makes living in defencelessness even more worthwhile.

So, the next time you find yourself fighting to be right, I

invite you to drop into your heart and release your need to be right. Look underneath to what is driving you and witness your own wound as you meet yourself with love first. Then turn that love outward and shine it on the other person. Be willing to see another perspective. Be willing to see their call for love and meet that call the best you can with as much love as you can possibly gather within yourself. Then watch the miracles unfold right before your eyes.

Day 13

What If Nothing Is Wrong? What If Everything Is Right?

Day 13 ~
What If Nothing Is Wrong? What If Everything Is Right?

Who decides what is wrong and what is right? Who passed the first judgment about wrong versus right? How do we really know something is wrong? How can we be sure something is right?

We go through life buying into the pre-programmed thoughts and beliefs that have been downloaded into our minds over the years. We are taught to respect our elders and persons of authority, and we start to believe them. At the same time, we stop trusting ourselves. We judge what happens in our life based on the filters in our own mind and the preconceived beliefs and opinions of society.

We can judge the divorce, the breakup, losing our wallet, losing our job, breaking our ankle, the devastation of a natural disaster, and all the other things that seem to be wrong.

But we also judge a new relationship, a new marriage, finding our wallet, getting a new job, being healthy, a hot sunny day, and all other things that seem to be right.

Depending on who is the judge and which filter we are processing our life through will depend on whether our minds deem those things as right or wrong. Who is the judge? Me? You? Society?

What if we have it all wrong? What if what we think is

wrong is actually right? How can we know for certain that what is wrong is wrong and what is right is right? We can judge what happens in our life as wrong, but what if everything is actually right?

A dear sister and friend from Cameroon, Jacky Essombe, told me a story once that changed my perspective and opened my mind forever. In a certain village in Africa the women would walk for miles every day to get fresh water for the village. It would take them hours and they would carry the heavy water containers back and forth every single day.

A humanitarian group came to visit the village and saw the long and tiring journey the women had to endure to deliver fresh water for everyone. They were moved to help. They arranged a meeting with the chief and elders—all men—and explained the time and energy it took the women to bring fresh water to the village each and every day. They offered to fund and build a well in the village so that everyone could access water without taking the long grueling journey through the hot sun to the current water source. The chief and elders agreed and the well was drilled.

Months later the humanitarian group members returned and were thrilled to see the well was providing a source of fresh and clean water to the entire village. They spoke to the women and expected to hear how happy they were not to have to make their long journey each day. To the surprise of the humanitarians, the women were not happy at all. They were disappointed.

It turns out they had enjoyed their walk each day. It had been a time for them to connect with each other, to laugh, sing, and tell stories. It was a sacred time that they had looked forward to every day. To the women of the village, the daily journey to get water had been a blessing. It had been a joy to spend time with their sisters and mothers. From their perspective nothing was wrong, everything was right.

The humanitarians realized that they had never asked the women if they wanted the well. They just assumed they would.

What if nothing is wrong in our lives? What if everything is right? What if we just need to look from a different perspective?

~

I am who I am today because of all those things going wrong and I am proud of who I am today. It is all a matter of perspective.

~

I can look back at my life and tell you many examples of things going wrong, doors closing, difficult challenges I had to face, obstacles that blocked my way, times when I was a victim of circumstances and bad things happened. Or I can look back on my life and tell you how all of those things shaped me, strengthened me, challenged me to change, opened my mind, broke open my heart, motivated me into inspired action, and gave me the courage to persevere. I am who I am today because of all those things and I am proud of who I am today. It is all a matter of perspective.

The truth is we can't get it wrong. Life happens and we deal with it in the best way we know how at the time. Sometimes how we deal with it brings us to our knees and we hit rock bottom and other times it lifts us up and builds strength and character. None of it is wrong. You can't get it wrong. That is good news.

Everything happens for a reason. In the middle of the chaos, the mess, or the life challenge, we don't always see why things happen as they do but we can all practise hindsight. I am sure you can look back at some things that happened in your past and find meaning and understanding that will help bring you peace.

~

The truth is we can't get it wrong. None of it is wrong. You can't get it wrong.

~

When I reflect on my miscarriage in 2001, I realize it was one of the most challenging and painful experiences of my life, but it was also one of the greatest gifts. Up until that point, I had been teetering between two worlds. It propelled me onto a beautiful new path in life where I would come to embrace my gifts as an intuitive healer. Without that experience, I wouldn't have started teaching Yoga for Fertility. I wouldn't have opened my mind-body studio or created my international Fertility Yoga Teacher Training program. I wouldn't have started communicating with spirit babies to connect parents with the child they are meant to welcome into their family. I wouldn't have learned to mother myself before my children came into my life. The list goes on. So many gifts came from that one messy life challenge.

Take a moment to reflect back on a past experience. Perhaps it is one you already made some peace around and you are open to finding a deeper meaning. It might be one that still haunts you with regret or heaviness.

Write down at least one thing you learned about yourself through that life experience. How did it strengthen you? Be open and curious. Chances are you will find more than just one thing. You can always continue to add to the list.

When we take the lessons from life and find the message

in our mess, we find meaning; when we find meaning, we find peace.

Now I will ask you one last time. What if nothing is wrong? What if everything is right?

I just explained how you can't get it wrong and that is true, but I have something else to share that might make your mind implode a bit.

You can't get it wrong and you can't get it right. It just is. Without judgment, life just is what it is.

~

Life just is what it is.

~

Stop judging life as wrong or right and instead trust that the unexplained circumstances are playing out for a higher purpose. You may not see the perfection playing out in the moment, but I assure you, if it is on your path, it is purposeful. The biggest source of suffering is caused when we resist life as it is. You can either resist it and judge it and cause yourself more suffering or you can accept it and embrace it and make peace with what is.

Life is just happening around us and how we respond to life will determine how we experience each moment. You can't get it wrong. You can't get it right. It just is.

Day 14

Everyone Makes Mistakes. Do We Judge or Forgive?

Day 14 ~
Everyone Makes Mistakes. Do We Judge or Forgive?

We all make mistakes and do things that can feel hurtful to others as well as to ourselves. When mistakes are used as lessons for learning, changing, and transforming, they can be powerful turning points. When mistakes are used to criticize, shame us, cast blame, and build a wall of regret, they become thorns in our mind; they just keep flaring up and blocking our ability to forgive ourselves and others as well as blocking our capacity to love.

When I felt the inspiration to write this chapter, I was very resistant to the topic I was shown to use as an example. I am going to tread softly and tenderly, but at the same time I know the topic is going to trigger some people. If that happens to be you, I encourage you to use the trigger as an opportunity to heal.

We are seeing a lot of women stepping out of hiding and shame and starting to publicly name and accuse men who have sexually abused or harassed them in the past. A courage is rising in all women to stand up, to be strong, and to be vulnerable as they tell their stories and expose the individuals involved. Some women are coming forward with secrets they have carried in shame for decades.

The #MeToo campaign that went viral in October 2017

with millions of tweets and Facebook posts within hours is a great example of women rising to tell their stories and send a message to men that sexual abuse is not okay. The number of responses is a testimony to just how many women have been affected and continue to be affected by unwelcome advances, sexual harassment, and/or acts of sexual abuse and violence by men.

First, I must say I am so sorry if it happened to you and I am sorry if you didn't feel like you could share what happened before now. I am sorry you had to keep the shameful event a secret for as long as you did. It happened to me too, more than once. In fact when the campaign went viral and my Facebook news feed filled up with women sharing their stories, it reminded me of other incidences in my life that I had buried in a dark hidden closet of my mind. The campaign has not only brought sexual abuse into the light of awareness to expose it and hopefully affect change, it has also provided us with an opportunity to heal our leftover shame, guilt, fear, and resentment around our own experiences.

Now here is where it gets a little sticky. It is true and I totally agree, it is not okay and it must be stopped. The question is how do we stop it? Is adding "shame on them" going to stop those men? For some it will. It will stop those who are just trying to fit in and go along with all the other guys. It may stop those who were only doing it because that is how they were taught to treat women based on the examples they witnessed. They probably already felt an underlying guilt about their actions. The campaign may cause tender compassionate men to stand up and stop another man from committing an act of sexual harassment or harm to a woman. I believe the campaign and women standing in solidarity are making a difference in many ways and I do encourage all of us to continue to rise up in courage and speak our truth.

My question is how do we stop it altogether? Like a weed that is pulled out without the root, this abuse will always grow back. How can we pull it out at the root so that the next generation of boys and men grow up with love, empathy, and compassion for women?

~

Before we can forgive, we need to feel all our unfelt feelings, cry our uncried tears, scream out our unexpressed words, and find loving supportive individuals who can hold space for us to process it all until we come to a place of softness and relief.

~

The difference between pulling the weed without the root and getting underneath it to the true issue lies in our own judgment and our choice to forgive. Before we can forgive, we need to feel all our unfelt feelings, cry our uncried tears, scream out our unexpressed words, and find loving supportive individuals who can hold space for us to process it all until we come to a place of softness and relief.

Next, the challenge is in letting go of our judgments of the accused men. Judging them will not help change them. There is a reason they commit these actions. It is a projection outward of their own underlying unresolved pain. There is an underlying fear that is driving their behaviour. Whether that be the fear of love, fear of rejection, fear of abandonment, fear of not having power, fear of feeling their own past pain and trauma, fear of their own memories of sexual abuse, fear of loneliness, fear of not being good enough, fear of looking like a fool .... I can go on and on and list all the possible fears that are the root that drives their behaviour, but it would take up most of this book. These men weren't born with these behaviours: they learned them and started using them as a way to cope with their underlying insecurities and fears.

Instead of facing their own internal demons, abusers project their unexpressed feelings out onto women and men through behaviours that help them feel better about themselves. The challenge is that they only feel better temporarily and an underlying guilt sinks in (with or without their conscious awareness) and they need to project again to feel better about themselves.

They don't need us to judge and shame them. That only adds to their underlying unfelt, unexpressed, unresolved root that drives their behaviour. Yes, the behaviour needs to be exposed and brought out into the light so they can't pretend and deny how they really feel underneath. But at that point, what they really need is compassion and support to help them heal their own internal demons and unresolved past trauma and fears. Once they own their part and take responsibility for their actions what they will need most is forgiveness. When they can genuinely and honestly say sorry for what they have done, we must forgive them. We must meet their fear with forgiveness and love and let love expand. If we do not, this cycle and unwelcomed behaviour will never end.

~

What abusers really need is compassion and support to help them heal their own internal demons and unresolved past trauma and fears. We must meet their fear with forgiveness and love and let love expand.

~

Now the more challenging scenario involves forgiving those who are not willing to apologize or own the harmful nature of their behaviour.

When I was in a counselling program learning how to provide support to clients who had been raped, someone asked the teacher if she had ever heard of someone being able to stop a rape as it was happening. She said in her experience, she had heard of two such examples. During the violent act, one woman looked deeply into the eyes of her rapist and genuinely and wholeheartedly said, "I forgive you." His eyes locked on hers and he felt her loving compassion and he immediately stopped and left her alone. Another woman had a similar experience and her words were "I love you." It wasn't about the words they used, but about the love and genuine forgiveness they felt as they spoke them.

Everyone makes mistakes. Some people make little ones while others make some big ones that impact many people. Forgiveness doesn't mean what they did was okay or right or acceptable. Forgiveness is always for ourselves first and foremost. Forgiveness frees us from all our resentment, fears, and trauma, and at the same time it just may have the potential to free another.

We all make mistakes. We don't need to be judged and shamed; we need to be forgiven and we need to forgive ourselves. Then and only then can we make a conscious choice for love and affect real long-lasting change on our planet. Forgiveness has the potential to heal humanity more than we realize.

Let's begin within our own hearts and minds. Who or what do you need to forgive?

Day 15

Stop Being Loyal

Day 15 ~
Stop Being Loyal

While most people believe being loyal is a good quality to have, loyalty actually stems from guilt, fear, and obligation.

We are taught that loyalty is an important quality to hold and something everyone should strive for. We are taught to be loyal to our friends and family. We are taught to be loyal to our country, our leaders, people of authority, and colleagues. We must be loyal. The message inherently also implies that if we are not loyal then we are disloyal, which can also translate to betrayal.

What does it really mean to be loyal? When we are loyal, is it acceptable to speak our truth when we have a different opinion? When we are practising loyalty, is there room to respectfully disagree with others you are expected to be loyal toward? Do we have the freedom to be ourselves or are we constantly striving to live up to the expectations of others to prove our loyalty?

~

Shifting from loyalty to people to honouring them feels more authentic and loving for everyone.

~

Loyalty is riddled with the ingredients of guilt, fear, and obligation. So how can we retranslate loyalty so that it feels more authentic and loving for everyone including us? We shift from loyalty to honouring.

I have supported hundreds of clients through healing displaced family loyalty. I had one client who was so loyal to his father that he gave up his career as a massage therapist to work as a roofer in the family business. He was experiencing lower back pain and together we discovered a growing underlying resentment buried under his allegiance and loyalty to honour his father's wishes. He hated roofing and didn't feel passionate about eventually running the family business. He loved massage therapy and helping others feel good in their body. After shifting from loyalty to honouring his father he finally was able to gather his courage to speak to his father and return to the career he loved.

A common pattern of displaced loyalty among my clients is a hidden block around abundance and success. We uncovered the belief that earning more income and becoming more successful than their parents, their siblings, and/or their friends was being disloyal. They would be stuck in a perpetual pattern of a drive for success followed by self-sabotage so that they wouldn't outshine their parents and perhaps make them feel bad.

So many people judge their parents for the job they did at raising them and then feel guilty about their judgment. Their loyalty runs deep enough that they find it hard to process their judgments without feeling bad. Loyalty keeps us trapped in the obligation to listen to and respect our parents; to take what they taught us and use it in our own lives. But what if what they taught us didn't resonate with us and we want to raise our kids and live our life another way? Would that mean we are being disloyal? Keep in mind most of this is going on behind the scenes in the recesses of our subconscious mind.

When I teach my clients to shift from feeling loyalty toward their parents to honouring them, their entire posture can change and their energy shifts from feeling trapped in guilt to feeling empowered with gratitude and appreciation.

Let's try it together. You can use this technique with anyone, but let's begin with your parents.

Take a moment to reflect back on the lessons, gems, insights, and gifts that one or both your parents taught you. Choose ones that you resonated with and appreciated. For some people, this will be easy and you will start a list. For others, you may need to take a different angle. Take some time to reflect and don't judge yourself if you can't find anything yet.

Now take a moment to reflect back on the things your parents did and what they taught you that you didn't like or agree with. Perhaps it was a technique for discipline or maybe they used negative feedback to motivate you. Be open and curious. Look back and ask yourself what that technique and feedback taught you. Maybe your parents' approach helped you get clear about how you would NOT want to raise your kids. In other words, you can look back and see what didn't work for you, which can lead to ideas and techniques that can work for you.

It is not about judging how they did it as good or bad or right or wrong. That is where feeling loyal to your parents will keep you stuck. Honouring them is about taking an honest look back and reflecting on how you felt, in order to get clear about how you would choose to respond differently today. You can also honour them for showing you how not to do it. It is not at all disrespectful; it actually fosters a genuine appreciation for the clarity you receive today.

It is important to take a moment to honour your parents for the fact that they really did the best they could, based on the circumstances and level of consciousness and awareness they had. They had their own triggers and reactions to parenting and most of them didn't know how to process their feelings. They did the best they could at the time. When you honour what you have learned from their actions and nonactions without judgment and you bring those gifts into your heart with gratitude, you are forgiving your underlying hidden resentment and leftovers to free yourself as well as them. Honouring is a gift for everyone.

Day 16

What Used to Work Is No Longer Working

Day 16 ~
What Used to Work Is No Longer Working

Have you noticed that what used to work is no longer working? Vices, substances, and tactics we used to use to distract, numb ourselves out, hide, and forget about our worries don't work anymore. While this may be frustrating or challenging for many because now they need to face all the feelings, traumas, and leftovers they have been avoiding for years, it is actually really good news.

We are all being called to do some spring cleaning, go through all the old boxes in our mind and body, throw out what is not useful or needed, and shift from living in fear to being in love with life. Those who are judging and resisting this process are feeling more intensity and pressure, and they are creating more pain and suffering.

The call to wake up and heal has become so strong that we can't avoid it any longer. When the call of our hearts was a whisper, we could pinch off the garden hose and stop it from flowing. We could use alcohol, drugs, exercise, food, TV, and other vices to detach from the underlying leftovers and ignore the call. Today, the call of the heart has become so strong, it is like trying to bend a fire hose to stop the flow of water. It is next to impossible.

Some people are still trying to avoid waking up, and the more they resist, the more painful it becomes. Many people are feeling so bad, they are projecting all their pain outward onto others in the form of violence, anger, and hatred. Many people are afraid we are going backwards and things are getting worse. Things are not getting worse, they are getting uncovered.

I worked with one particular client for a few years and I kept getting the message she needed to quit drinking alcohol. In the beginning, her body would react to alcohol with specific symptoms but she would ignore them and convince herself they were related to food or something else. At the same time, her guilt was eating away at her insides because she knew on a very deep level that her relationship to alcohol was not healthy and that she was meant to quit drinking alcohol altogether. She continued to ignore the message and she resisted for a long time. Her symptoms got worse and worse. Her resistance to quitting drinking showed up as a desperate quest for answers to her health issues. She would jump from doctor to doctor hoping for answers to her health issues.

Each time we would join for an intuitive reading, I would receive the same message for her to quit drinking alcohol. She didn't want to hear that answer. She resisted for a long time, until finally at one point she agreed to stop drinking for a period of time. Her physical symptoms improved dramatically and some of her health issues went away completely for months. Slowly, after a period of time they started to return. She would bring them to our session with confusion, worry, and desperation to find an answer. I kept being pointed back to alcohol, but I thought she had quit drinking until one day I asked her straight out, "Are you drinking alcohol again?" It turns out she started having the occasional glass of wine with dinner around the same time the symptoms came back.

She was so resistant, convincing herself there was something else going on that she didn't see the connection and timing of reintroducing alcohol to her diet and her body's negative reactions.

I helped her see how she was using alcohol to self-soothe—as a way to avoid feeling some underlying emotional pain and past trauma. For years, alcohol was working to calm her mind and keep her past emotional trauma hidden away. It was clear the message was getting stronger and stronger and at the same time her resistance was growing stronger and stronger, until finally she hit a wall and had a breakdown. It was in that moment that everything shifted and her mind opened up to the truth that alcohol was no longer calming her but was creating chaos on every level, including physically and emotionally. She finally agreed to quit drinking the second time and face the inner demons that had been haunting her for years. Her physical symptoms improved and many disappeared. As she continued to heal, feel her feelings fully, and integrate some healthy tools to calm her mind, her whole life shifted. She started to process her daily life triggers with awareness and intention, and her health continued to improve. She felt a renewed sense of purpose and experienced deep authentic peace.

~

People are no longer able to hide their opinions, judgments, and beliefs. It is all coming out into the open.

~

All the darkness that we thought was gone is actually lying dormant, hidden in the shadows. At this time, everything is coming out into the light. People are no longer able to hide their opinions, judgments, and beliefs. It is all coming out into the open. People are even taking off their masks and marching outwardly and openly showing what they stand for. This is good news. As long as people hold onto those hidden thoughts and beliefs, they remain in the dark corners away from the potential for healing.

Some intense dark programming is surfacing and coming into the light for healing. As a lightworker and healer, my role is to bear witness to it, make a conscious choice for love, and take inspired action only. If we add our own fear to the fear, fear expands. When we meet fear with love, love expands. Now that doesn't mean we sit back and do nothing. Some of us will be called to stand and speak up. Others will bear witness. Others will become fierce loving warriors facing the fear head on. We all have roles to play. When we let our heart lead, we will get clear about what our particular role is. We are only meant to play our part, however big or small that role seems. Each role is essential to the healing of the whole of humanity.

We are all being called to surrender and let our hearts lead the way. In order to do that, we need to be willing to let go of control and drop into trust. We need to be willing to feel the old dense emotions we collected and buried over our lives in order to free ourselves from them once and for all.

~

We usually heal in layers.

~

The good news is that it doesn't happen all at once. We usually heal in layers. Yes, some layers will be dense and intense, and for many it will take courage, but all of it will rise up for healing whether we want it to or not. We are coming to a point when it is becoming non-negotiable. We can process our leftovers, move through our fear and resistance, and align with our heart's path, or we can prolong our suffering and it will continue to grow in intensity.

We can either embrace healing or resist it. We still have the right to choose but the consequences of resisting it are powerfully intense. The good news is the rewards of embracing healing are extraordinary and full of miracles. The challenge comes in the process of embracing it—we need to move through the phase of unwinding our minds, letting go of our judgments, facing our fears, feeling our emotional density, and clearing a path to love. Depending on how much avoidance one practised and how much emotion one buried will determine how challenging the process may or may not be. For some, it will be a walk in the park; for others it will be like walking through a mucky swamp.

We are not meant to do this alone. Asking for help and being open to support from others will quicken the process and provide a gentler path. Having compassionate witnesses will help us heal some of our deeper wounds with less suffering. Our ego mind loves to create more suffering and make things harder than they are meant to be. While I am not saying it will be easy, I know we all have the capacity to stop hiding behind our vices and take steps to awaken to our fullest potential.

I have explained to many of my clients and my Heart Led Living community members that it used to be much harder to be awake in this world. It was easier to sleep walk through life. Now the time has come when it is much harder to stay sleep walking than it is to awaken. I know we can all do this. Each one of us can awaken to our full potential and inspire others to do the same, creating a beautiful ripple effect that will touch the hearts of all of humanity. We can do this! I have complete faith in every single one of us!

Are you willing to feel to heal?

Are you ready to let go of what is no longer useful or helpful?

Are you ready to face your fear and resistance head-on so you can free yourself?

Are you willing to say YES to life and start living your full potential?

Are you willing to play your part?

I have complete faith in you! You are ready! And the world is ready for you!

Day 17

Stop Taking Everything So Personally

Day 17 ~
Stop Taking Everything So Personally

When we stop taking everything so personally, we free ourselves from judgment and suffering, and open ourselves up to experience acceptance, peace, and compassion.

We have been taught to judge ourselves and others so much that when others don't do what we think they should do, we take it personally. We have become so personally invested in what others say or do that we feel a sense of responsibility; we believe their actions reflect on who we are. We have gotten so wound up in what others are doing, we can't see that it really has nothing to do with us. We get caught up in a grey area that keeps us whirling in projection, guilt, resentment, and blame.

~

What others do or don't do is not about you: it is about them. How you feel and your judgments about what they do or don't do are about you. When we can separate our stuff from their stuff, we can actually heal what is underneath.

~

What others do or don't do is not about you: it is about them. How you feel and your judgments about what they do or don't do are about you. When we can separate our stuff from their stuff, we can actually heal what is underneath. As long as we take it personally, we will use projection as a way to keep us from owning our own stuff and we won't be able to heal it. As long as we project and blame someone else for how we feel, we will be stuck in helplessness disguised as resentment. Our potential for healing the root of our upset will remain hidden to us. Through projection we throw our own stuff onto someone else and it ends up being out of reach of our awareness. We are too busy blaming another to look within and realize it is our own trigger we need to heal.

It is helpful to embrace the idea that our triggers are opportunities to heal some underlying leftover trauma, pain, or limited belief. People just do what they do and sometimes what they do doesn't bother us and sometimes it does. When we feel triggered, that indicates that life is bumping up against something we need to heal. Triggers can be embraced when we intentionally use them for our healing. Triggers cause more suffering when we don't.

I am one of those people who shows up on time and I prefer to be at least ten to fifteen minutes early. Being on time generally comes naturally for me. In the past, when I was late for an appointment or a meeting I would beat myself up about it and feel extremely guilty for keeping someone else waiting. I would feel bad and blame myself even if it was due to circumstances that were out of my control.

When other people showed up late, I was over-the-top accommodating and accepting because I didn't want them to feel bad or guilty. I valued being a people pleaser more than I valued my own time spent waiting for them.

I noticed with one particular person when it happened more than once that she showed up late, that I started to feel more and more restless and triggered. Every time we would set up a time, I would already assume she would show up late, but I never said anything. I started to feel anxious and resentful watching the clock; then she would finally show up. All the while, I never said anything; but my resentment was growing.

My ego would jump in with thoughts like, "She is taking advantage of you. You should really say something. Don't let her walk all over you like that. She is disrespectful and rude." I started to explore my inner dialogue and feelings of resentment. I was doing okay until one day that person didn't show up at all. I waited an hour or more and I was fuming, shaking, and over-the-top angry. When I got home, I sat on the couch and sank into all that I was feeling. It was as though a volcano had erupted and I felt out of control.

The longer I sat with my feelings the deeper I went, and I had this flash of all the memories of the times I spent sitting at our front window waiting for my dad to come pick us up. I would show up early and wait for hours. Most times, he showed up, but a few times he didn't come at all. Those were painful experiences because I only saw my dad once or twice a year. I longed to see him more and each time I was told he was coming, I was so excited and I anticipated his visit often by counting down the days, hours, and minutes. When he didn't show or he was late, I was always afraid he wasn't going to show; my heart felt bruised, heavy, and sad.

A layer of deep sadness washed over me and I cried all my uncried tears. I felt a sense of loss, of missing out and, at the same time, of yearning for his love and attention. After a few hours, I started to feel lighter and compassion entered my heart. I knew he had struggled to see us. I knew it wasn't easy for him. I knew he had a lot of fears he wasn't willing to face. I knew he did the best he could, given the circumstances. I for-gave him. I for-gave myself. I for-gave my mom. I for-gave everything over for healing and I made a conscious choice for peace.

Then I brought my attention back to how I felt about the individual who didn't show up for our appointment. I felt compassion. I felt for-giveness. I felt peace. I saw the gift that came from my willingness to look within and face my own trigger. It wasn't really about them. It was about how I felt about them not showing up or being late. By shifting from taking it personally and feeling angry to owning my own trigger, I healed a huge layer of childhood trauma. I felt gratitude toward her.

As I took some time to reflect, I realized that this person was chronically late for everything. It wasn't just about me and her being late for the appointments she booked with me—she was always late, always apologizing, and always repeating the same pattern with everyone. When I took a step back and wasn't taking her behaviour personally, I could see that she was just doing what she always did. When I brought that awareness back to how I feel about her always being late, I recognized a pattern in me. I was a chronic accommodator and people pleaser who wasn't willing to say anything when other people were late for fear of making them feel bad. The other piece I saw was by behaving that way, I was dishonouring myself and disrespecting my own time. So I decided I would say something, not because she needed to change, but because I needed to set a healthy boundary to honour myself and my time.

I was clear and concise when we spoke, because I had no judgment and I had already cleared my own trigger. I explained that I needed to set a healthy boundary to honour my own time and she understood. She shared how she felt when she was chronically late and I shared a few suggestions that would help her break her habit. Although I wasn't attached to any outcome during our conversation, something shifted and she was never late for any of our appointments after that. I felt a sense of peace and joy for our exchange and the miracles that followed. My courage to look within and explore my own triggers led to a healing for both of us. I started to look at my triggers as beautiful hand-delivered messengers disguised as life's circumstances.

The next time you take something personally, be willing to stop and explore how you feel. We are never upset for the reason we think. Let your judgments go and look beneath them for the root of your trigger. You may be surprised by where it leads you. There will be times when you will be guided to say something and set a boundary, and there will be times when you won't. Trust your heart to lead you. In the meantime, use your triggers as opportunities to heal any leftover trauma and free yourself from the buried ongoing suffering. Then celebrate the miracles and open your heart to return to peace, love, and compassion.

Day 18

Pain Is Not Our Enemy but Our Ally

Day 18 ~
Pain Is Not Our Enemy but Our Ally

When we learn to embrace pain it becomes our greatest ally, a friend pointing to what we need to see in order to move beyond it. We are taught to try to move away from, avoid, or numb our pain. We take a pill, have a drink, distract ourselves, or ignore it. We are programmed to believe that pain is our enemy and we need something external to help alleviate it.

Pain is a signal from our body asking us to pay attention and telling us where to look. Every time we try to numb it out or ignore it, we are attempting to turn off the signal. In a sense, we are saying no to the message the body is holding for us, as well as to the potential for healing.

Pain can come in the form of a physical sensation in our body, looping self-defeating and limiting thoughts, or emotional trauma, or intensity and stress. It is a signal that something is not in harmony and needs our attention and awareness. I teach others to bring their awareness toward the source of their pain so they can receive the message and do what is necessary to bring the body back into harmony. I have worked with clients who have had chronic pain for years; after one session it is gone. When we get to the root of the pain we can heal it at the source.

Sometimes, our pain is simply unfelt emotions accumulating in one area of our body. For example all our uncried tears and unexpressed grief and loss can be stored in our lungs. Resentment is often stored in our liver and/or in our hips. Fear can often be found accumulated in our kidneys or upper abdomen. Our psoas muscle, which runs from the inner thigh, through the pelvis and attaches along the surface of the lumbar vertebrae, is a muscle that holds the energy of panic and fear.

~

Something as simple as changing our thoughts about pain while we are experiencing it will reduce suffering.

~

When we are willing to go into our pain and explore it with a curious nonjudgmental mindset we can actually gain some incredible insight that often leads to miraculous healings. Sometimes we can do that on our own and at other times we need some support. Some of our wounds need witnesses and they will require more courage to explore. In those cases, it is helpful to have a guide or to work with someone who can help us through the process. This can be essential, especially when exploring pain we have been avoiding for so long that it becomes difficult to get through the thick layer of fear on our own.

Exploring our emotional pain is just as important as exploring our physical pain. I have had many clients during healing sessions suddenly feel sad but they aren't sure why. They hold back the tears in embarrassment or out of the habit of holding onto their emotions and judging them, especially when they have no obvious reason to be sad. When I tell them it is okay to be sad and I give them permission to cry, they break down and release a flood of tears. Once the tears stop flowing, they feel relief and often experience a sense of peace.

Most of the time, our emotional pain just needs an outlet and it will rise up and out to be released. Emotions are meant to be felt, expressed, and released, but we tend to judge them, hold them in, or resist them, especially when we can't pinpoint what they are related to. Sometimes we will just have a wave of emotion rise up that isn't directly connected to the present moment. If we can allow space for the emotion to move through us, we can process it more quickly than if we question or resist it.

Our minds are programmed to add more suffering as we move through pain. We use the word "pain" to label a lot of physical sensations and negative emotions. The word "pain" has a lot of meaning tied to it and a lot of history and fear associated with it. If we use other words to describe the sensations and feelings, we can soften our experience of the pain. Using words like "dense, tingling, throbbing, pulsing" or describing the size, shape, and colour of the area can help us explore it through observation instead of with judgment and fear. As we shift our thoughts and judgments around pain, our experience of pain shifts as well.

Something as simple as changing our thoughts about the pain while we are experiencing it will reduce suffering. Our own thoughts can increase or decrease our suffering. If our thoughts play into our being a victim of our pain, we will feel more like an out-of-control victim and we will suffer. Our own thoughts can even increase our pain instantly. When we change our thoughts, we can move from being a victim of our pain to being a curious observer. This opens our mind to a whole new level of awareness and insight and it softens our experience.

In the beginning of my pregnancy with my son, I was terrified to have any pain or sensation I didn't understand. I was afraid for the first five months because I had had a previous miscarriage and it took two years to conceive again. The miscarriage itself had been excruciatingly painful as I ended up with an infection and I had to have two surgeries. I went through a lot of emotional and physical pain. My mind was set on the belief that I was a victim of my circumstances. Yes, the physical pain was intense and I suffered a lot. In hindsight, I see how much my own thoughts added to my experience of the pain and contributed to my suffering.

In the last four months of my second pregnancy, I was practising yoga, meditation, and other relaxation techniques to prepare for the delivery. I still had fear because I always joked that I have sensitive pain receptors. I didn't know how I was going to handle labour pain. One of the biggest things that helped was stopping people who wanted to share awful stories about births going wrong. That was not helpful at all, so I would interrupt people and say, "I am not interested in hearing any negative stories, thank you." My own thoughts were enough to deal with. I didn't need more evidence from others about how I might not be able to handle it and what might go wrong. I turned my focus inward onto my own thoughts.

At the thirty-two-week mark of my pregnancy, I had just finished teaching a cardio core class and I started to feel some intense cramping. I sat down in the office and put my head down on the desk. I stopped my thoughts from reeling in fear and calmed my mind. I started to explore the sensations and bring my awareness right into them. I was witnessing, feeling, sensing, and experiencing without thought, fear, or worry. I was a silent observer, fully present with my breath and the sensations. I was fascinated by everything and I didn't feel pain—only waves of tightening then softening. Then my thoughts began and I felt the intensity increase and it became more painful as worry filled my mind. What if something is wrong? Am I going into labour early? This can't be good. Just as I was about to call for help, everything stopped.

About a week later, I felt the sensations start again. This time I was in bed with my husband beside me. I stopped my thoughts and calmed my mind. I brought my awareness into the physical experience and started to witness the sensations. My mind remained quiet as I was deeply present with my breath and my body. I allowed no thoughts to enter my mind. It was peaceful and at the same time the sensations were strong enough to capture all my attention. After what felt like about five minutes, the sensations ended as suddenly as they had begun. I opened my eyes and looked at my husband. He told me I had been in that state of deep relaxation for about thirty minutes. What I thought was only five minutes was actually thirty. That gave me the confidence that I would be able to handle my delivery and birth.

During my labour, I was in that same deep state of observation without thoughts. I was calm, my mind was quiet, and I had my own internal world of observing every sensation. I was deeply present with my eyes closed the entire time. There were only two moments I remember having a thought enter my mind. One was around the eight-hour mark, when I realized it was dark outside. I could feel an undertone of suffering as I tried to figure out how long it had been and how much longer it would take. The sensations intensified as I asked my doula, "How much longer?" Her response was, "One breath at a time" and everything softened and I sank back into my internal world of observation. The second thought came later as a fleeting thought of compassion: "I understand why some women would ask for an epidural." That thought left creating no change in my sensations. I can see in hindsight how my first thought—the one of suffering—caused my body to tense and

I felt more pain. The compassionate thought that came later had no impact on my body and in some ways it helped me surrender even more.

Now I know some of you will enjoy that story or feel neutral when you read it, while others may be triggered by it. I am not saying all women will experience a pain-free labour. That was my experience and each person's experience will be different. I am simply sharing an example from my life about how my own thoughts of suffering created the experience of increased pain for me. If you are triggered by my story that may be an indication you have some leftover trauma held inside that is rising up for healing. I would encourage you to reach out for help so you can heal it and free yourself.

Here is a process that can provide support as we explore pain in our body and open up to receive a message.

1. Find a comfortable position and close your eyes.
2. Take five deep breaths.
3. Let go of everything you think you know and everything you think you don't know about your pain. This will create an open and curious mindset to explore the pain.
4. Imagine you could bring a light of awareness and shine it on the area of pain.
5. Start to find any words to describe it (for example, its size, shape, colour, sensation, density, and location). It is helpful to move away from the label of "pain" or "painful."
6. As you explore the area of discomfort, be wide open to any messages in the form of words, images, memories, colours, or insights.
7. If there are any emotions present, create space for the expression of the feelings as they arise. Cry any tears, feel the anger, or allow the natural release of the emotion

in whatever ways feel natural at the time. Emotions are energy in motion. When we allow the emotion to be expressed in whatever way it needs, we are letting the energy move up and out of our body and freeing ourselves from it. The challenge is that many people judge or avoid their emotions, especially emotional pains. This causes unprocessed emotions to be stored as dense energy that blocks their systems leading to dis-ease. I always teach others to be willing to "feel it to heal it."

8. Imagine you could for-give everything and place it on a healing plate in front of you. Imagine through your offering you could release it from your body and ask for healing.

9. Be open and curious about any guiding steps that will help you receive a full-circle healing around this area. For example, you may feel guided to journal, reach out for support, see a doctor or practitioner, or take a hot bath. Let your body lead you to what you need when you need it. Your body wants to return to harmony and it knows what it needs and when. Trust your body and its innate wisdom to heal.

As we embrace the idea that pain is not our enemy but a signal from our body to pay attention and look within, we can use it to heal what is hidden. I often tell my clients I go through the body as a doorway to heal the mind. I use the body and any sensations or discomfort as entry points to trace the signal back to its root. So I invite you to be open and curious to explore what it might be trying to tell you, the next time you experience any pain. Use the process above and if you still need support be sure to reach out and ask for help. Some of our wounds need witnesses for us to heal them.

Day 19

There Is What We *Want* to Hear and What We *Need* to Hear

Day 19 ~
There Is What We *Want* to Hear and What We *Need* to Hear

I always tell my clients, "I won't tell you what you *want* to hear, but I promise to tell you what you *need* to hear." Sometimes what we want to hear is what we need to hear but more often than not, what we want to hear is nowhere near what we need to hear. There are two ways to do it: either with judgment, criticism, and blame or with fierce love, compassion, and grace. I choose the latter.

It is not always easy to tell others what they need to hear, but my clients come to me because they want to see their blind spots and heal what is hidden so they can change what is no longer working in their life. They respect my level of raw vulnerability and tell-it-like-it-is approach. They are grateful for my radical honesty. I will tell them what others won't, because I want them to heal their unhealthy patterns and be better versions of themselves. We can't see the picture when we are in the frame and so we need others to tell us what we need to hear.

Recently I was supporting one of my clients through a challenging situation with her father. He has remarried and his new wife is extremely controlling and manipulative. When my client's father's health started to decline, she felt compelled to stick up for her father by talking to his wife but the message

I received for my client was quite the opposite. I kept hearing the words: "His relationship is none of your business." We discussed how his relationship was his choice and, at this point, she wasn't meant to interfere. She had to take a step back and let go of her own fears in order to find a way to support him without imposing on him her judgments and opinions about his relationship. She needed to focus on being radically honest with herself before she could be present for her father in a loving supportive way.

There is a big difference between brutal honesty and radical honesty.

~

Brutal honesty is insensitive and often delivered with an intention to hurt, shame, or blame someone. Radical honesty on the other hand is delivered with love, compassion, and tenderness.

~

Brutal honesty is insensitive and often delivered with an intention to hurt, shame, or blame someone. Radical honesty on the other hand is delivered with love, compassion, and tenderness. It holds the intention of supporting the other person to increase their awareness around what they need to change, to help them take an honest look at themselves, and to make a conscious choice to shift their behaviour and mindset so they can become the best version of themselves. We tell them what they need to hear because we love them enough to be honest. Even if what they need to hear won't necessarily feel good, we know it is purposeful for them to heal and make a conscious choice to change.

Unfortunately we are taught if we don't have anything nice

to say then we shouldn't say anything at all. We are taught to bite our tongue and not rock the boat. It is true sometimes we are meant to remain silent and mind our own business; there are also times when we are meant to stand up and speak our truth but we are afraid to do so. We are afraid we might hurt someone's feelings, others might disagree with us, we might be judged by others, or we might be attacked and ridiculed. There are so many more reasons to stay silent these days, but what the world needs is for everyone to stand up and speak their truth.

Now I can pretty much guarantee when you speak your truth that you are going to be judged, so you can just accept that fate right here and now. Social media has become a battle ground of judgment. It seems to be a damned-if-you-do-damned-if-you-don't arena. The virtual distance gives people courage to publicly criticize, judge, and be downright mean. We have come to a point when it doesn't matter what we say—people will judge us. Even when we remain silent, people will judge us. It doesn't matter whose side you are on or what opinion you hold—I promise you there will be someone who will pass judgment. That is the result of our fear-based programming.

The good news is that when you say what you are meant to say it will have an impact on those who are meant to hear it. Let the judgers judge. They are not your intended audience. If they are going to judge anyway, you might as well give them something worthy of their judgment. Now that we have that all clarified and we know what to expect from the judgers, let's talk about the impact we can have on those who are meant to hear our message.

Have you ever looked in the mirror and discovered you had spinach stuck in your front teeth? Why did no one tell you? They felt uncomfortable and didn't want to embarrass you so they just let you go through your day for hours with a green leaf in your teeth. How is that supportive, loving, or helpful? As uncomfortable as it might be, I do my best to let people know when they have food in their teeth, their bra is showing, they tucked their skirt in their pantyhose, or they have toilet paper stuck to their shoe. I would want someone to tell me, so I assume most other people would want to know.

There are times when we will see someone behaving a certain way and we may notice how their behaviour impacts those around them. Most times they are not aware of how they are being perceived by others. We may feel compelled to tell them and we can do so with the intention of creating awareness so they can make a conscious choice to change. Remember to come from a place of fierce love, compassion, and grace. Now I need to be clear—it is not about being nice. It may not sound nice but it is necessary.

I often say to my clients, "This may feel sharp or thorny," because I am radically honest with them. They may or may not accept what I have to say and that is okay. They may be triggered or get upset at first and that is okay. As long as I come from an intention of loving guidance I know I am playing my part. What they do with it will be up to them.

More and more people are speaking up and sharing messages that the world needs to hear. It is and will continue to be uncomfortable for many but, in order for everyone to heal, we need to be willing to take a good honest look at everything including how our own behaviours impact others. As I explained on Day 2 in "We Are More Connected Than We Are Separate," the sum of the parts contributes to the healing of the whole. Each human being in their own unique way is contributing to the healing of the whole of humanity. We each need to be willing to play our part.

Some of us are being called to say things that are

controversial, uncomfortable to hear, and may uncover and stir up the past, but that is what is necessary in order to impact change on a global scale. Some of us will play an essential role in calling people on their stuff and shaking things up so others can wake up. We each need to take a good honest look at how we are contributing to the behaviours that lead to our demise and how we are contributing to the healing that we all need as a species.

There is a powerful call to heal ourselves and our planet. We are each being faced with a courageous choice to do what we know we are meant to do. Many of us will need to forgive and everyone will need to make a conscious choice for love.

The time is now. No more delay. Say what you are meant to say because there are people in the world who need to hear what you have to say, in your way with your voice. There are people who will only hear you. There may be some who don't want to hear it, but they still need to hear it in order for all of us to create the quantum shift on our planet from fear into love. All I ask is that you play your part; however big or small it is, your part is essential.

Day 20

**A Living Breathing Classroom
Designed Just for You**

Day 20 ~
A Living Breathing Classroom Designed Just for You

Our life is designed perfectly for us. Our environment, relationships, experiences, obstacles, challenges, miracles—everything is being beautifully orchestrated for us to heal all our fears and overcome all our limitations. We are each meant to become a full expression of our truest self so we can love deeply, impact change, and uplift humanity. We do that by following the breadcrumbs life places on our path.

We are programmed to believe that life is happening to us, that we are always victims of a series of random circumstance that we have absolutely no control over. This is still the mindset of about eighty to ninety percent of the population. This keeps us in a loop of grasping desperately for some sense of control only to spiral further into helplessness and defeat. For some, this mindset brings a drive for power.

The power I am referring to is superiority power with the intention of exerting control over others. These power positions are all ego-feeding fear-based approaches that make the controller feel powerful but can cause a lot of pain and suffering for others as history has proved over and over again.

Feeling like a victim can bring about feelings of blame, anger, resentment, and even violence. People who feel like victims react to life with fear, confusion, and uncertainty in a desperate attempt to regain a sense of control and power. They believe that if they can change the circumstances, change their life, or change others, they will feel better. They believe life needs to change before they can change. As long as they hold the mindset that life is happening to them, they will always feel like victims in any and all circumstances.

When we shift from "life is happening to me" to a new perspective that "life is happening for me," we can shift from feeling like a victim to realizing that we have the ability to enhance our experience of life based on how we choose to see life's circumstances. Life still happens, but our response to it shifts. We no longer react to life, we respond to life with curiosity about the twists and turns. We trust that in some way or another, everything is playing out purposefully just for us. We can find meaning and empowerment and a sense of purpose. Challenges become choices to respond to with love or fear. Obstacles become opportunities in disguise. We are participating with life as our classroom for creating awareness and healing our minds.

Now, if we take this viewpoint to another level and shift our perspective to "life is happening through me," we will recognize we are actually the captain of our own ship, the director of the play, the teacher who is on some level creating the curriculum in our unique life classroom. Our life is responding to how we feel, what we believe, and the way we respond in each moment. If we live in fear, we attract more experiences that keep us feeling afraid. If we expect miracles, we attract and experience more miracles. We now realize we have the ability to create our life with intention. We have the power to change our circumstances based on how we feel, what we think, and what we desire. As long as our desires are in alignment with what we believe, we can manifest the life of our dreams.

~

If we live in fear, we attract more experiences that keep us feeling afraid. If we expect miracles, we attract and experience more miracles.

~

Now bear with me as I take this a step further. Some will be ready to embrace this or may already be living from this place, but most of the population is living somewhere within the previous perspectives. This may or may not be a stretch for you but surrender everything you think you know and imagine your mind is wide open. How do you feel when you try on these words? "I am one with life, life is one with me." From this perspective we are living oneness and bypassing the limited potential of our mind to tap into a force within us that has direct access to a field of unlimited possibility. We come to realize we are actually creating as ONE with our Soul, our Source, our God, the Universe, the Divine; use whatever word resonates at the deepest level of your being. We open our minds fully and surrender our plan and our will; we make a conscious choice to embrace the grand plan.

When we let our heart and souls take the lead, our lives change in an instant and the side effect is an abundance of miracles. We experience a deep sense of peace, knowing, and trust. We no longer react to life; we embrace every aspect, knowing it is all purposeful. Every moment becomes a gift that we unwrap with great anticipation for the miracle it holds. We feel a sense of oneness with our true Self, each other, and our planet. We can see ourselves in each other and each other in ourselves. We are united in love and we feel whole and complete.

In one of my recent weekly Heart Led Living Community

calls, I encouraged my members to approach Christmas and the holiday season with the intention to heal. I asked them to use the holidays and family gatherings as a classroom and to be open to any and all opportunities to create awareness and heal their family triggers and leftovers. I will invite you to do the same during any upcoming events in your life. By watching our own thoughts of judgment, fear, and worry, and at the same time giving ourselves permission to feel our feelings, we can shift old patterns and potentially heal them for good.

One of my clients is working on stopping her pattern of people pleasing and putting others' desires ahead of her own. It has been a sticky process of unwinding old family patterns and she is saying no more often. This is triggering other family members, because she is standing up for herself for the first time and it is uncomfortable for everyone. At the same time she is feeling more and more empowered and seeing the miracles that come from trusting and following her heart.

I use every moment of my life as a classroom to heal, grow, and evolve. I use every trigger or upset to get underneath it to its root and I unwind my mind to align with love. It requires a conscious choice to be wide open to another perspective and to take a radically honest look at our lives and our relationships.

~

I unwind my mind to align with love.

~

In every moment, we have the choice to challenge our current thoughts and try on another perspective. Where do you stand on these four different ways of living life? Remember your intention is to create awareness without judgment.

1. "Life is happening to me ~ I am a victim of life's circumstances." These people are still asleep to the potential life holds. The key elements to make the shift in this phase are awareness and acceptance.

2. "Life is happening for me ~ I am starting to wake up to see that life is our classroom." These people are feeling empowered with potential. The key elements to make the shift into this phase are faith and forgiveness.

3. "Life is happening through me ~ I am becoming more aware of how I am creating and using my life to heal and embrace conscious living." The key elements to make the shift into this phase are trust and curiosity.

4. "I am one with life, life is one with me ~ I am living Oneness." These people feel connected with all that is. They feel united in love for self and others as well as for our planet and beyond. The key elements to make the shift into this phase are surrender and love.

Once you are aware of where you are living your life, there is always an invitation to shift your belief and try on another perspective. Take your time and use each stage for your own healing. Most of us are not meant to skip a level or take a quantum leap from victim to oneness. It is too much for the programmed mind to authentically embrace. Most people find purpose moving through the stages as they unwind their mind, heal the leftovers from their past, and gradually come to embrace a new way of being.

Honour the stage you are in and be open to a shift. Be patient. This chapter has planted the seed of possibility. Trust your life classroom to provide the curriculum you need to heal, grow, and expand. Follow the breadcrumbs. Be willing to use every experience for your deepest healing so you can fully awaken without any leftovers. Trust your life to unfold as it is meant to unfold. Your life is a classroom designed just for you.

Day 21

Saying No Is Saying YES

Day 21 ~
Saying No Is Saying YES

When we say yes when we actually want to say no, it is more of a disservice to everyone including ourselves. I will say that again in another way: if you say yes when you are meant to say no, you are stealing the opportunity from the person who is actually meant to say yes, and you are denying yourself an opportunity to say yes to something else that is meant for you.

How many times have you said yes to someone when you really didn't want to? Many people say yes to avoid disappointing others. They say yes because they are afraid to let others down. If you have a hard time saying no or feel super uneasy when you do, I guarantee you have a bad case of people pleasing. Stop people pleasing. It is not helpful, because it stems from a place of guilt, fear, and/or obligation.

~

If you have a hard time saying no or feel super uneasy when you do, I guarantee you have a bad case of people pleasing. Stop people pleasing.

~

Many people have such a hard time saying no that they believe it is just easier to say yes. That may feel true in the moment perhaps, but in the end, they tend to overcommit themselves, which leads to burnout, resentment, and regret.

Saying no is not always easy, especially in the beginning, but it is necessary if you want to do what is right by everyone. It starts with being willing to practise saying no when you mean no. Saying no is the best gift you can give yourself and others. Saying no allows you to say yes to what you are meant to say yes to. It frees your time and energy for the things you are truly meant to focus on. Also when you say no it creates space for others who are meant to say yes.

I used to have such a hard time saying no. I was extremely uncomfortable with no. I am a recovering people pleaser. I have gathered some tools and a new perspective that have helped me shift my experience of saying no from feeling bad to feeling empowered.

Here are some tips that may help you to say no more comfortably.

1. Just say no without any excuse, story, or reason: When we justify and explain ourselves we are not standing solid in our decision to say no. We are waffling and people pleasing, trying to explain why we can't. It also opens up space for the other person to talk us out of saying no and persuade us with creative solutions so we can say yes. For example if I say, "I am sorry I can't help out; I need to pick up my daughter at that time," it gives the other person the invitation to try and help you find a solution. They might say, "You can ask your husband to pick her up or I could pick her up instead. That way you can be there." If you just say, "No, that doesn't work for me" or "No, I am not available," that will close the door on any potential negotiations. If they try to persuade you anyway, just repeat the same words: "No, that doesn't work for me." You will feel tempted

to say more; don't do it. Trust me—after a few times of saying it, you will feel more empowered and there will be less guilt.

2. If it is not an absolute heart YES, it is a no. I get asked to do a lot of different things and some stuff sounds like it would be really fun to do, but I only say yes to the absolute heart YESes. That preserves my time and energy for what I am really meant to be doing. Saying yes can come from one of two places—our heart or our head. Often when we are saying yes from our head, we are either people pleasing and feel guilty and obligated or we are basing the decision on some other fear (consciously or subconsciously). When we feel a heart yes, it is coming from a place of love. When we let our heart lead, saying yes is an act of love for self and others. We are following that inner knowing that is operating on behalf of everyone. When our head is in alignment with our heart, it makes the choice much easier. A heart yes is a feeling of expansion, light, or peace within. A heart no is a feeling of tension, heaviness, or discord within. When we say no because our heart says no, we are making the choice that is for everyone's highest good, even if that means disappointing someone. It is not always comfortable but there are powerful lessons in it for everyone when we learn to listen to our heart and say no when we are meant to say no and yes when we are meant to say yes.

3. Buy yourself some time. You don't need to say no right on the spot. If you are tempted to say yes and feel pressured to give an answer right away, buy yourself some time. Let them know you will check your schedule and get back to them or that you will call them back in

five minutes or the next day. Buying yourself some time gives you an opportunity to check in and make sure it is a clear heart no. It will also give you time to stand solid in your heart's true answer.

4. Saying no is a yes in disguise. When we say no to something we are saying yes to something else. Saying no is actually honouring and creating space for our heart's YESes. Saying no is a gift for everyone including yourself. The next time you say no, ask yourself, "By saying no right now, what am I actually saying yes to?" This turns your attention away from the energy of no and potential guilt and brings your awareness toward the yes energy so you can expand in excitement and anticipation.

5. Practise hindsight and expect miracles. In the beginning, it may help if we practise hindsight and pay attention to how things play out when we do say no. Perhaps there was someone else who stepped up to the plate and said yes or the person asking you to do something found another creative solution. Perhaps the project shifted directions altogether and something new and more expansive was born out of it. Be curious and be open to the miracles that come after you say no; they will enforce your faith in following your heart.

Here is just one of the many examples of the gift that came when I followed my heart to say no. I was asked to speak at an event scheduled in May 2015. After tuning into my heart, I received a no. I didn't understand why, because the event sounded really awesome, but I have learned to trust and follow my heart's guidance; so I said no. It turns out that year in May I took my first humanitarian trip to Africa. On the day of the event, I wasn't speaking on stage in a beautiful venue; I was walking through the sewage-filled streets of one of the largest slums in Kenya, empowering the women and children. It was one of the most powerful eye-opening experiences of my life. The trip also fulfilled my life long vision and a deep heart calling to travel to Africa to be of service and provide support. I was able to touch the hearts of many women and feel the children's joy despite how little they had. My heart was forever changed and my Heart Led Living Foundation was born.

We don't always know at the time why we are guided to say no, but as we learn to walk with blind faith, we can trust we are saying yes to potential miracles.

The next time you are faced with a decision and you feel like saying no, just do it. It may feel uncomfortable at first but that is only because it is unfamiliar. It will get easier as you practise, especially if you pay attention to the miracles that come when you trust and follow. Your heart's YESes are gifts for everyone including yourself. You will come to honour and cherish the noes, because you know in your heart they are truly gifts in disguise leading you to miracles that your mind can't even begin to imagine.

Day 22

Embodying Your Heart YES

Day 22 ~
Embodying Your Heart YES

If everyone stopped focusing on the noes in their life and brought all of their energy and attention to the YESes, their entire outlook and experience of life would change in an instant. When we focus on the no, the door that is closing, the relationship that is dissolving, or on any resistance we have to how life is playing out, we will feel stuck, disconnected, and a victim of life's circumstances. When we embrace and embody our YES for life we will feel empowered, excited, and alive with unbridled enthusiasm and anticipation for all that life has to offer.

The first step is to stop focusing on what isn't working and isn't coming together as we had planned in our heads. Life has a way of directing us. As one door closes, there is always another one opening. We may not see it right away and if we are staring at the closed door asking why, we may never turn around to find the other doorway all lit up and open for us. Focusing on the no keeps us in a victim mindset feeling like a victim of life's circumstances. It is that mentality that life is happening *to* me that I explained in "A Living Breathing Classroom Designed Just for You." As long as we keep our attention on the no, we will not be open to a creative solution, a life redirection, or a new and exciting adventure. Focusing on the noes leads to more noes, which leads to self-defeating behaviours and deflating and debilitating experiences.

When we place our attention and intention on how life is saying YES to lead and direct us in our lives, we will experience deep peace, extraordinary joy, abundant miracles, and exciting adventures. Our heart's YES is a signal that we are on track, living our purpose, and fulfilling our destiny. From our human perspective, we don't always see the perfection playing out, but we can trust it is all playing out for everyone's highest good including ours.

It is essential we learn to discern between a true heart YES and our head's version of yes. Our head's yes is based on logic and reason, either weighing the pro and cons or deciding based on what we think is best for us and others. It is a limited-perspective yes that is based on our limited thinking mind. Our truest heart's YES is based on a higher perspective, one that only our Soul has access to. Our heart bridges our human perspective with one that is being operated and orchestrated based on the needs of the whole of humanity and our planet. Our deepest desire is to follow our heart YESes, because we know they will lead us to the path we are meant to walk and ultimately allow us to play our part to uplift humanity and unify us in love for each other and our planet.

~

Our deepest desire is to follow our heart YESes, because we know they will lead us to the path we are meant to walk and ultimately allow us to play our part to uplift humanity and unify us in love for each other and our planet.

~

Our heart's YES is actually humanity's YES.

So how do we discern between our head yes and our true heart YES? It is about getting out of our head and into our heart and feeling into every decision from that deep place of knowing. Our heart YES will likely feel light, expansive, open, and soft; it may feel like a smile inside your heart. It can be one or a combination of all these feelings. It may help to feel the contrast of your heart NO, which feels more tense, heavy, tight, constricting, and closed, and you may even feel yourself cringing inside.

It can vary for people, so it is important not to compare and judge how you feel your heart YES with how someone else experiences it. As you practise discerning your own heart YES, you will get clearer about how it feels for you and it will become more natural to identify and follow it. Once we get a clear experience of how our heart YES feels in our body, we can use our feelings as signals to light our path and direct our decisions.

The next step is to embody our YES for life. This morning I woke up and took a moment to say YES to all that life has to offer me today. I invited the feeling of YES into my heart and then into my entire body. I felt a softening, an opening, and a willingness to embrace all the gifts that life will deliver to me today. I know that some gifts will come as opportunities disguised as challenges. In fact, I take moments throughout my day every day to embody my YES.

I trust that all of life's circumstances are designed to direct me and are part of the grand plan. When I start my day feeling a YES for life, I align with divine strength and courage that carry me through every moment and they open my heart and mind to experience more joy, happiness, and peace. I am wide open to see the miracles as they are unfolding and I set an intention to celebrate each one. Since I learned to intentionally embody my YES for life every day, my life has expanded in ways that I couldn't have imagined.

My heart is more open to receive my husband's unconditional love; my relationship with my body and my health has improved dramatically, and I feel more alive than ever before; I have healed my money blocks and opened my life to receive abundance and prosperity; my business is evolving and growing in creative and exciting ways; and my life is flowing with beautiful ease and grace. Yes, I still face challenges like everyone else, but I don't resist anything and my response to life embodies the energy of YES! This allows me to accept, surrender, embrace, and navigate life in ways that allow me to remain at peace with all that is and be wide open to all that is possible.

The part I am meant to play is shifting, expanding, and evolving, because I am surrendering and allowing life to unfold for me, through me, and as me. I am answering my calling to play bigger than ever before, to create even greater impact, and to empower millions of people. I can feel it in my bones. My life's purpose and my entire being are evolving. The time is NOW. There is no more delay. I say YES to my heart's call. I say YES to play my part. I say YES to what my soul is wanting to birth through me. I say YES to my gifts and to sharing them on global stages. I say YES to all that I am meant to be, do, and have. I am ready and the world is ready for me, whether it likes it or not, whether it knows it or not; it doesn't matter, because I KNOW it and I say YES.

Now it is your turn.

Begin with identifying, feeling and discerning your heart YES. Then surrender your plan and align with your heart's plan. Let your YES expand beyond your heart and feel it in every cell of your body. Imagine it taking up all the space within and around you. Fully embody the feeling of YES, YES, YES for life! Imagine softening and opening your heart wide to receive all the gifts that life has to offer. Life is full of opportunities to heal, to expand our minds, and to align with love. It is full of exciting adventure, heart-touching moments, tenderness, extraordinary acts of love, and enormous abundance. It has so much to offer all of us. Will you say YES and unwrap the gift of each present moment with great anticipation? Are you ready to embody your YES?

Say YES.

Just say YES!

Day 23

When We Take Things Way Too Seriously

Day 23 ~
When We Take Things Way Too Seriously

Many people take life way too seriously creating way more pain and suffering for themselves. Yes, stuff happens, the shift hits the fan, but we don't have to let the tough stuff take us down. We can use our life to empower ourselves and lift us up. It all begins within our own mind.

If we pay any attention to the news today, we can gather much fear-based evidence that the world is going to crap. And if our minds are open, we can also find just as much evidence that the tides are turning in the direction that is allowing an evolution of love, hope, and inspiration. What you focus your attention on expands. If you focus on the bad, you will see more bad. If you focus on the good, you will witness more acts of love.

When we take things too seriously, it is hard to see any perspective other than the bad. It is like wearing a shade of sunglasses that only sees all the problems. When we are feeling heavy and serious about all the problems, we are not open to tapping into the potential for creative solutions.

The emotional vibration of seriousness is very low, heavy, and dense. It is not a fun place to camp out in and we are not fun to be around. There is no potential for joy, happiness, and play. There is barely any room for love.

When I was growing up I always took life too seriously.

In recent years, I have named one of my ego personas "Serious Sue." She is a great worrier. She knows how to find something—anything—to stress about. When I became a mother, "Serious Sue" became a strong contender for leading my life. My playfulness was present when I sang to my son, but as he grew older I grew more and more serious.

One day, I was half joking about my serious side and how it has taken over my life when someone asked me, "Why are you so serious?" It was such a powerful moment because I had never asked myself what was behind my drive to be serious. So I embarked on a journey of self-inquiry and jumped in with a full commitment to get to the root of my seriousness.

I spent time journaling, I did a worry-free-week exercise, I meditated, I practised laughing yoga. I did anything and everything I could think of to get underneath my seriousness. Finally, through authentic journaling, I received some insight. Authentic journaling is a channeled conversation with my higher Self. I start out the journal entry with, "Dear Self." I take a moment of gratitude for the connection and open my heart and mind for guidance. I ask questions and receive answers.

When I asked, "What is the hidden belief that is the driving force behind my seriousness?" the answer came through words onto the pages as plain as day. "The world is a painful place. It is not safe and you need to protect yourself and everyone else." My son and daughter came into my awareness and I felt a fierce "mother bear" protective energy rising up. It was in my chest and back. My teeth and jaw clenched tight. My hands went to fists ready to fight and defend. I felt a raw intense rage rise up like a bubbling volcano ready to explode.

My natural desire to protect and help others was completely infected with a worldly threat of war. I witnessed it all, I felt the energy coursing through me, and I surrendered to the emotional roller-coaster that followed. I had visions and memories and flashes of images all showing the evidence of just how unsafe this world is and how much pain it causes. It took a while to process and eventually it calmed down and my body softened.

As I lay on the floor with tears flowing, I vowed to see another perspective. I vowed to see a world of love, compassion, and safety. It was in that moment the root and the driver of my seriousness cleared. Now when "Serious Sue" shows up, it is easier to identify, change my thoughts, shift my perspective, and lighten my mood. She doesn't have a strong life-threatening hold on me anymore. I can see it is only the habitual mind bringing "Serious Sue" into the mix and I have a choice to give her space to worry or to dismiss her with love. I have a deep sense of peace and calm inside and out. There is more space in my mind and heart to laugh more and I feel lighter each day as I continue to invite playfulness and fun back into my life.

My fear about the world being unsafe and full of pain was a subconscious program that had been driving my behaviour since childhood. Once I uncovered that, my experience of life changed.

~

It is not about what is happening but about how you choose to feel about what is happening.

~

So the next time you feel yourself getting too serious, be willing to look underneath your behaviour and be open to see what is driving you. It is not about what is happening but about how you choose to feel about what is happening. That choice is either conscious or subconscious. As you soften your mind and open your heart to discover what is hidden underneath, you are making a choice for conscious change. Be patient. Be willing. Be curious. You never know what you can uncover and the freedom that is possible when you do.

Day 24

All Relationships Will Either Evolve or Dissolve

Day 24 ~
All Relationships Will Either Evolve or Dissolve

We have come to a time when all relationships need to be re-evaluated. We need to take an inventory of which relationships are helpful and which ones are hurtful. Which relationships lift us up and which ones tear us down. Some relationships are meant to be released so they can naturally dissolve, and others are being called to evolve. These relationships may be with parents, children, siblings, friends, partners, business colleagues, and professional clients. Practising discernment and non-attachment is essential in creating awareness as well as in reducing the suffering that can go along with this process.

You may have heard the saying, "People come into your life for a reason, a season, or a lifetime." It is true: some people are meant to play a bigger role in our lives while others teach us what we need to learn and off they go.

The challenge comes in our judgments about who is meant to come and who is meant to stay. Many people are so loyal to family that they are not willing to consider they are meant to let go of a relationship with a family member or a spouse or a partner. Instead of letting go, they hang on for dear life and create way more suffering. I have seen it over and over again with clients who hang on to relationships and marriages that are meant to end. Eventually they do end. Many times, some people need to stay in longer just to make sure or to feel like they have tried everything before they give up.

Remember on Day 5 how I shared my reluctance to end my relationship with my boyfriend in "What We Can't See, We Can't Change"? It is very common to hang on longer than we are meant to. Letting go of a relationship that is meant to end is not giving up—it is accepting the inevitable. Now, let me be crystal clear. It is not wrong or a bad thing to stay in a relationship longer because you want to be sure or to feel good about knowing you did everything you could to see if it could evolve. All I am encouraging everyone to do is start to identify which relationships are meant to dissolve and to let them go sooner than later.

Having said that, some of us will still need to learn our lessons the hard way and that is okay. Those hard lessons are powerful teachers. I have learned many of my most powerful life lessons that way. I have now come to a place in my life when I no longer wish to inflict more suffering. I also have a deeper trust in my ability to discern. I have been practising non-attachment for years now. Letting go has become easier for me. Relationships are more challenging but with continued practice and awareness, I am gaining confidence.

~

When it is time to let go of someone, our attachment may stop us from seeing how the relationship is not serving us anymore.

~

When it is time to let go of someone, our attachment may stop us from seeing how the relationship is not serving us anymore. We can attach ourselves to individuals themselves or to the dream of what we thought the relationship would be like. We can be attached to objects, places, and experiences we associate with the person, we can be attached to hopes that it will change, and we can be attached to dreams and visions of the future. Attachment can prevent us from letting go and cause us to hang on so tightly that we end up being dragged along, creating way more pain and suffering in the process.

Not all relationships are meant to last a lifetime. When we accept that some people will come into our life for a reason or a season, we can allow the organic progression of each relationship to play out. When it has taught us what we need to learn, we can allow the relationship to dissolve. We can consciously let go and make peace. It may take a long time to process some relationships.

With every letting go, there is often a sense of loss. With letting go of some people, we will feel the loss and process it with ease; with others, it may take us some time to grieve. It is helpful to reflect on what we learned from being in each relationship. Take all the gifts, lessons, and insights you gained and bring them into your heart with gratitude. Feel any feelings of loss and imagine yourself freeing the other person and yourself, so you can both move on. Sometimes we can look back in hindsight and find meaning as we see the perfection of how it all played out. Other times, we just need to trust it wasn't meant to be. In both cases we can let go and let be.

I can think back to relationships I had in school. On graduation day, we all promised to keep in touch. There was an anticipation of what was next for all of us and at the same time a letting go with a sense of loss. After graduation, I never heard from some of those friends again. Some of those lost friendships have been rekindled through Facebook. I did stay in contact with some of my friends from school and when we get together or reconnect, it is as though no time has passed.

When a relationship comes to a point where it has been maximized, meaning it has taught us everything it can possibly teach us, it will either dissolve or evolve. Letting go of relationships is one thing that can be very challenging, but evolving relationships can be just as challenging if not more so. When a relationship is being called to evolve it takes great courage and willingness from both sides to take an honest look at what is working, what is not, and what needs to change in order to allow for its evolution.

~

Letting go of relationships is one thing that can be very challenging, but evolving relationships can be just as challenging if not more so.

~

When I started questioning my own marriage, I was relearning how to build my business without pushing myself so hard that I would crash over and over again. It was a fine dance between inspired action and deep rest and rejuvenation. I was learning how to fill my heart first and give from the overflow. My spiritual practice included yoga, meditation, reading, studying, and vibrant self-care. I was discovering a way to shift from hard work to heart work. I felt like the foundation of who I was in the world was shifting at a very deep level.

At the same time that I was personally evolving, I felt disconnected from my husband. It was like we were going on with our day-to-day family stuff as roommates living under the same roof. It was like I was living in two different worlds: my heart work, which was my soul-enriching work, and my relationship, which was feeling stalled and stuck in old patterns and repetitive issues looping over and over again. I felt as though I had changed and evolved personally but our relationship hadn't. Something needed to change.

One night while my husband and I were going through the motions of our nightly family routine, I decided I had had enough. I gathered up my courage to open a conversation and share how I was feeling. I knew he was feeling the disconnect as well, but he didn't know how much it was dragging me down this time. There was too much of a contrast between how I was being in the world and how I was living at home.

We talked for a few hours as I explained that I couldn't keep doing this. I was tired of the old pattern playing out again and again and again. I told him that our relationship either needed to evolve or I needed to leave. We had very different views on life when it came to our beliefs. I had strong spiritual beliefs and a clear purpose in life. He wasn't interested in my spiritual practices or beliefs. He respected mine but he wasn't interested in embracing any of it for himself. It felt like we were at a standstill. Heart Led Living was my life, my purpose, my soul's path, my every moment, and my every breath; I needed to be able to bring it home. Although he always let his heart and intuition lead him, he wasn't interested in taking the same spiritual path I took.

Faced with the idea that my marriage might be over, I started to explore my attachments to everything including him. I imagined my life without him. I reflected on how I would feel, what my life would look like, where I would live, how that would change life for my children. I explored all of it fully until I exhausted all my attachments and I felt open to what was meant to be.

One day when I was speaking with my dear soul sister and intuitive counsellor Rev. Lisa Windsor, I shared my fear that my marriage might be over. I talked about how different my husband's and my beliefs were and how I needed a spiritual practice within my marriage to support its evolution but my husband didn't resonate with my current practice and didn't feel that he should have to change his beliefs to match mine. He was right and I understood. He was standing up for his beliefs and I was standing strong in mine. I needed to find a way to bridge the gap between us or it would be over. Lisa suggested, "Radical honesty." The words jumped into my heart and I felt a huge surge of energy. YES! That feels good.

When I shared the idea of our spiritual practice within our marriage being a practice of radical honesty, my husband said, "I can do that!"

I took a deep breath of relief and gratitude for finding some middle ground that could honour both of us. We started a radical honesty practice every night before bed. We also started to be honest throughout the day and share things that trigger us and also share things that we are grateful for. Our connection grew deeper and stronger than ever before. We were connecting and sharing deeply, and he was sharing more honestly and not holding back. We shared our deepest hidden fears. We shared our needs and desires. It was not easy. It was the most challenging time for both of us as we exposed all the things we had been holding back to clear any and all underlying resentment, hidden thoughts, and deepest desires.

My husband and I are solid today and continue to practise radical honesty especially when we start to let life get in the way of feeling connected. I gave myself permission to start being more authentic and speaking my spiritual language in our home openly and honestly. I gave myself permission to be myself and I gave him permission to be himself. It was so freeing. After sixteen years together, we are more in love than ever before. I can say without a shadow of a doubt that the practice of radical honesty saved my marriage and I am deeply grateful for both our courage and our willingness to evolve our relationship in a way that we both felt and still feel honours and respects us.

Take some time to reflect on all your relationships and be open, honest, and willing to explore each one. Some will be obvious, while with others you will need to take some time and maybe a radical honest conversation to get clear about them. Some relationships will need to dissolve or perhaps they already are organically dissolving. In that case, your intention is to release any attachments and let them go. Some relationships may have already evolved without your realizing it. Celebrate those and honour the gifts and lessons that they continue to extend.

The relationships that need to evolve may be your most challenging work ahead, but I assure you it will all be worth it. An evolved relationship is a powerful, supportive, and loving relationship that can carry you through so much. We often have evolved relationships with the people who come into our life for a lifetime; these are essential relationships that support our life's work and purpose.

If you need support and feel inspired to start a radical honesty practice, you can tune into my radio show episode where I explain how to begin. Many couples have listened to the episode and started their own practice to support the evolution of their marriage. You can tune in here: heartledliving.com/radical-honesty-saved-my-marriage.

I will leave you with one other idea. I have mentioned that all relationships need to evolve or dissolve and I mean all relationships, including the one you have with your Self. Practising radical honesty with yourself is powerful and transformational. The world needs you to evolve and answer the call in your heart. We need you to be a full expression of YOU unapologetically. That requires you taking a good honest look at what behaviours, beliefs, fears, and patterns are blocking you from shining your brightest light, living your best life, and being your most authentic expression of YOU. Are you ready to evolve and answer the call of your heart? Say YES! Just say YES and watch the miracles unfold.

Day 25

What We Seek from Others, We Must First Give Ourselves

Day 25 ~
What We Seek from Others, We Must First Give Ourselves

Many people are desperately seeking something, anything, and everything from others. They are either trying to fill the void or emptiness they feel inside, or they believe that there is something outside themselves that will provide the answer to their problems and make them feel whole again. Seeking ends up being a wild goose chase that will keep them running in circles, never finding what they really need. They may find what they think they want, here and there, but they will never find what they need.

What we seek from others we must first give ourselves. When I first heard these words, I felt a deep surrender, my shoulders softened, and I experienced a huge relief. I didn't realize just how much pressure I had placed on myself to find the answers to all of my life's problems externally. All my life I was a perpetual seeker of knowledge and understanding. I was not only constantly seeking information but I was always secretly seeking the Truth. Why am I here? What is all this for? Who am I really?

My natural tendency to seek information outside myself grew and became quite unhealthy in many ways. One of those ways was seeking love and acceptance from others. I wanted everyone to accept me, to like me, and if possible to love me. I wanted so badly to be loved because I didn't love myself. After an incident of sexual abuse at the age of five or six years old, I shamed, blamed, and shunned myself. I decided I deserved to be punished and I wasn't worthy of love.

Having that deep-rooted subconscious belief made it challenging growing up, because it was in direct conflict with my seeking to be loved. Even when love was expressed toward me, I found it uncomfortable to accept and sometimes I didn't even recognize it as an expression of love. I was seeking love but didn't know how to receive love or recognize it.

When I started to try on the idea that what we seek we must first give ourselves, it was around the time I was in an intensive three-month counselling training. We covered content like sexual abuse and trauma and other sensitive topics. A lot of healing occurred for me during that time. My husband and I had only been together for about a year and were not yet married. I was practising opening my heart to let in the intensity of his love for me. My heart would open for a few hours, for a few days if I was lucky, then it would slam back shut.

I started to play with the idea of seeking. Every day I would ask myself, "What am I seeking?" Each day I would get a piece of the puzzle and I would take that information and turn it inward toward myself. The first day I started to explore this, I noticed that when I sneezed, my fiancé (at the time) didn't say, "Bless you." I had noticed it before and was often a little disappointed because he was so attentive and loving in every other way. Why did it bother me so much that he didn't say, "Bless you"?

My ego mind would have dismissed it, but I was really curious. I was seeking a blessing from him, so I turned it back onto myself. If I can't get it from him, I will give it to myself.

So the next time I sneezed I said, "Bless Sue" out loud and I giggled. It felt so good. It felt light, peaceful, nurturing, and at the same time really playful. Something shifted and I no longer felt I needed a blessing from him because I had already given it to myself.

~

What we seek, we must first give ourselves. So I turned what I was seeking back onto myself. Something shifted and I no longer felt I needed a blessing from him because I had already given it to myself.

~

Within a few more times of me blessing myself after sneezing, my husband started saying, "Bless you." When I was no longer seeking it from him, the gift was extended. When I no longer needed it to fill the void, it came with sincerity and love without my even asking. What a gift.

Then I noticed he started waiting and not saying "Bless you" after my first sneeze, so I asked curiously why he paused to say it. He said, "Because you always sneeze in twos, so I wait until after your sneezes are finished." Bless his sweet soul.

Another lesson I used this tool with was seeking love. I turned that back onto myself and started extending love toward myself from myself. I used to hate myself, especially throughout my time with anorexia and bulimia and alcohol and substance abuse. At first, sending love to myself was uncomfortable and awkward. It felt like a lie, but I kept going, convinced that I was no longer going to seek love outside myself and was determined to give myself all the love I could ever need or want.

After about six months, my affirmations in the mirror and all my intense healing work finally paid off. Something shifted deep inside and I started to feel more authentic in the love I extended toward myself. I shifted from self-hatred to self-love. Now, I can say I love myself. I honour my needs and make my self-care a priority. I have learned to fill my heart first and give from the overflow. I have learned to mother myself so I can mother others without self-sacrifice. I have come a long way using such simple words to turn it all around.

What are you seeking?

What do you think you need from others?

What void or emptiness are you trying to fill by seeking something outside yourself?

Are you willing to turn it around and start giving yourself what you are seeking and be open to a shift?

Be curious. Be open. Be willing to see the truth so you can set yourself free. Whatever you seek, turn and give it to yourself; open your heart wide to receive. It will be one of the best gifts you will ever give yourself.

Day 26

I Know Nothing About Anything

Day 26 ~
I Know Nothing About Anything

When we finally embrace the truth that we know nothing about anything, we will find true freedom and our lives will expand in ways we could never have imagined. So much emphasis has been placed on knowledge that we end up filling our heads with too much stuff. We are taught to make decisions based on logic and reason. We are encouraged to think about it and weigh the pros and cons before we make any decision. What if we are going about it completely the wrong way?

There is knowledge that we gather in our head and there is knowing that resides in our heart. We have been taught that knowledge is more important than knowing. The knowing in our heart goes beyond the physical limitations of our mind. It is a knowing that taps into a source that is acting on behalf of everyone including you. When we align with the knowing in our heart, we are opening up to a network that connects us all and is being orchestrated for all of humanity and our planet.

~

When we align with the knowing in our heart, we are opening up to a network that connects us all and is being orchestrated for all of humanity and our planet.

~

Our mind thinks it knows but our heart knows. Our heart bridges our limited human perspective with the field of pure potential. Have you ever had a knowing that goes beyond all logic and reason? Have you ever just known something and you couldn't explain why? This is the knowing I am referring to. We each have access to it but most of us are so busy living in our head that we don't tap into the wisdom and knowing in our heart. Our head overrides anything from our heart. We think we know better because we are taught to lead with our head and not trust our heart.

We have it all backwards. We are meant to lead with our heart. We are meant to use our intuition as an internal guidance system. Our heart is meant to be in the driver's seat and our head is to be used as a tool. As Albert Einstein said, "The intuitive heart is a sacred gift and the rational mind is a faithful servant. We have created a society that honors the servant and has forgotten the gift."

The biggest block for many people is that they think they know what they don't know. Our mind thinks it knows because we have gained knowledge, but our mind holds such a limited perspective and potential. Knowledge is not knowing. So how do we get out of our head and into our heart to tap into the infinite knowing? We can begin with admitting that we know nothing about anything.

In my book *Heart Led Living ~ When Hard Work Becomes Heart Work*, one of the ten principles that helps us lead with our heart is "Be Curious." When I first heard the words "I don't know and it's okay," I was baffled, because I tried to wrap my head around it and at the same time I felt an underlying sense of peace. I sat with the words for weeks reflecting on the idea that I don't know. "I don't know and it's okay" was the first step to accepting the truth. Then came "I don't know and I am curious." Curiosity created an opening in my mind and allowed me to at least listen to what my heart had to say. The next step was "I don't know and I am glad." There was a great relief and freedom that came when I no longer had to figure everything out. It was comforting to know my heart would lead me for every decision and every step.

Recently in meditation I received the words, "I know nothing about anything." When I took the words into my head to grasp an understanding, I spiralled into confusion, but suddenly everything softened and my mind was incredibly quiet. "I know nothing about anything" brought a deep sense of peace because I didn't need my head to know anything. It was as though my mind had emptied everything out leaving infinite space. It was nothing, yet at the same time it was everything. I saw my mind held nothing and my heart could access everything. The knowledge in my head emptied and my heart filled up with a knowing that came with no words or knowledge, a knowing that was unexplainable, a knowing that could only be experienced. It has left me with a feeling I still can't explain in words.

When we can embrace the idea that we know nothing about anything, we open our minds up to receive directions from an all-knowing, all-seeing source that is acting on behalf of everyone, everywhere, all at once. We can bypass our limited minds and bridge the gap between what our mind thinks and what our heart knows.

Now here is another stretch for your thinking mind. What if our mind was not actually in our head? Yes, our physical brain is in our head; but what if our mind wasn't just in our head? Be curious and open as we try on this idea together.

There is our thinking mind, which I like to refer to as our head, and there is our whole mind that resides in every cell of our body. We think our mind is in our head because we use the cells in our brain to think with, so the mind feels activated and concentrated there. Just for fun, imagine for a moment that your mind was not just in your head but it was in every cell of your body. As you bring your awareness down into your body, imagine that you could activate and wake up the mind in every cell. Close your eyes and notice how you feel in your body and if you feel any different in your head. Take some time with this exercise.

When I take my clients through this guided exercise, most experience a feeling of expansion in the mind and a relief of pressure in their head. There is often a sense of calm and lightness that follows.

We are so used to concentrating our efforts and using our mind's limited capacity, because we think it is in our head. So we are essentially only activating our mind in the cells of our brain. When we allow our mind to be activated in every cell of our body, we are expanding our capacity and getting out of our limited thinking mind and aligning with our whole mind.

One thing I know for certain is that I know nothing about anything. I am not even attached to any of these words or ideas in this book. They are simple words and ideas that are purposeful to help open our minds to another possibility. They are designed to unwind our limited thinking minds to create an opening and try on another perspective. They are purposeful until they aren't. For whom and how they are purposeful are none of my business. I am simply the channel to allow the words to flow through. They are all coming from the knowing that I can access through my heart. I am simply the messenger for the message at this time.

We are each messengers in our own unique ways. When we accept that we know nothing about anything, a beautiful gift for humanity will come through us. Each of us has an essential role to play. Are you willing to let go of everything you think you know and let your heart lead the way? Are you willing to shift out of your head and into the infinite wisdom of your heart to sing the song you are meant to sing, to write the book that you are meant to write, to innovate and create a vision that only you can deliver to the world?

We are all waiting for you to say yes with great anticipation of the contribution you are to make to uplift humanity. Let's all say yes together.

Day 27

Dying to Feel Alive

Day 27 ~
Dying to Feel Alive

Many people die having never truly lived. They spend their life slowly dying and missing out on the experience of ever truly feeling alive. Our deepest desire is to feel alive with purpose and passion. We are meant to leave this Earth feeling like we made a contribution. We each have a unique gift, talent, or legacy we are meant to bring, share, and extend to others in our lifetime. When we remain blind to our contribution, we spend our life dying to feel alive.

My deepest desire and purpose is to not only leave the world a better place than I found it; I have a grand dream, a huge calling to contribute to transforming it altogether. My biggest dream as a child was to save the world, as I've said. It was grand, it was exciting, it was exhilarating, and it made me feel alive. I felt empowered until gradually my ego mind took hold of that dream and it became painful, heavy with responsibility, and a huge burden to bear, especially for a little girl.

I was dying to live my dream but my ego convinced me it was impossible. I lived many years with that deep desire constantly calling me and at the same time I was haunted by my cruel destructive inner dialogue.

"There is no way one person can save the world."

"Who do you think you are?"

"You don't even deserve to be alive."

"No one loves you."

"You might as well be dead; you are never going to amount to anything."

"Give up and die already."

In spite of my inner demon, I still followed my desire to help others, nurture animals, and do my part to preserve nature. Eventually I had to let go of my dream to save the world, because I started being attached to other people changing their ways or wanting to heal them. Some people were willing whereas others were not. I focused on those I couldn't save and I carried that until it became a burden. I felt deeply hurt when others didn't care about animals, nature, and the planet the way I do. It devastated me and I lost hope once again. But again that calling inside me persisted, so I decided that I couldn't let those who didn't want my help to stop me.

After years of therapy, using mind-body techniques, energy healing, coaching, and my sheer determination to heal anything and everything that was standing in the way of my dream, I realigned with it. I had a renewed sense of hope that I could help those who were willing to accept my help; I could become a partner and guide on their healing journey; I found my sense of purpose and passion again. I was thriving and I built my own business around it. I was living in my own little world, creating impact, seeing the transformation of my clients and community members, and celebrating the miracles in every moment.

As I started writing this book, that big grand dream to save the world came calling once again. Yes, I was already making a difference in the lives of thousands of people, but I knew in my heart I have a bigger part to play. I have something more to contribute and it is time to step up to the plate and breathe life back into my grandest dream to save the world.

In this moment when I reflect on the words "save the world," I feel differently about them. I feel empowered. I feel a realm of possibility. The energy behind the words has changed for me in the process of writing this book. It is no longer based on fear and needing to rescue everyone along with all the animals and the planet. No one needs rescuing; they need to feel empowered to fulfil their purpose and answer the call of their heart. It is not about the words "save the world." It is about the feeling I feel behind those words and the meaning I place on them now. For me, they capture the essence of waking up the world.

~

Now, the words "save the world" capture the essence of waking up the world.

~

I am connected to a deep knowing in my heart and soul that I am ready and the world is ready for me. All I need to do is play my part in the grand plan and support others to do the same. I know in my heart that I can "save the world," but I don't need to do it alone. We are not meant to. When we combine each of our dreams, they lead us to a shared vision to leave the world a better place than we found it. We are each meant to make our unique contribution as well as a collective contribution that has the embedded potential to transform the world altogether.

Some of us have a big part to play. I have come to embrace that I am one of those people. It used to terrify me; now it drives me, it thrills me; the idea makes me feel alive in a way I have never felt before. I feel deep peace, extraordinary joy, and unbridled enthusiasm for life and what is possible for all of humanity and our planet.

I feel I can step into my full potential, share my contribution to the world, and play my part in my dream to save the world. One day, I will die knowing that I left no stone unturned, I played full out, I put all my cards on the table, and I extended all that I had to give to leave a legacy of love. Our dreams are actually drivers that ignite our passion, our creativity, our love, our light, our essence. It is not about the end of the dream and whether it came to fruition or not—it is about feeling alive in every moment and enjoying the ride we call life as we embody the essence of potential within our dream.

~

Our dreams are actually drivers that ignite our passion, our creativity, our love, our light, our essence.

~

I will end with one of my favourite quotes by Howard Thurman. "Don't ask what the world needs. Ask what makes you come alive, and go do it. Because what the world needs is people who have come alive."

Take some time and reflect on the following questions. First close your eyes and imagine dropping your awareness down into your heart. As you ask the questions, allow the answers to pop into your awareness. Go with the first answer, to start your exploration.

What's your dream?

What have you always wanted but have been too afraid to do?

What are you most passionate about?

What brings you joy?

How are you meant to contribute to this beautiful world?

What makes you come alive?

All it takes is a moment of courage to say YES to giving your dream space to come alive. Your dream contains your unique contribution. Your part is essential. The world needs you now more than ever!

Day 28

When You Resist Life, Life Resists You

Day 28 ~
When You Resist Life, Life Resists You

When we look around at our planet, everything appears to be falling apart at once. Many people are afraid we are going backwards, but the truth is everything is getting uncovered, coming into the light of awareness, and rising up to the surface for healing. The world is being called to awaken all at once. This is the most powerful call for love that has ever existed. We have two choices: either resist and suffer or surrender our fears, embrace life, and say YES to play our part in the grand plan to awaken our planet.

With all that is going on in the world, we can find a huge list of reasons to resist life, to be afraid, to hide, to avoid, and to duck and cover. It appears as though life is throwing every opportunity it can to challenge us to the core of our being. Even Mother Earth is discharging a large amount of accumulated energy through hurricanes, earthquakes, fires, volcanoes, and storms. Mother Earth is not angry; she is healing and she needs our support not our fear. The call to heal and transform our planet has never been more powerful and the call continues to get stronger and stronger every day. The more we resist the call in our heart, the greater resistance we will encounter.

Answering the call is non-negotiable. It is inevitable. So how do we begin within ourselves, in our own lives, to release our resistance and embrace the healing transformation that is occurring all around us? We first need to change our perspective about what is happening at this time on our beautiful planet.

~

So how do we begin within ourselves, in our own lives, to release our resistance and embrace the healing transformation that is occurring all around us?

~

First, let me be clear—we are not going backwards and we are not losing ground. It is quite the opposite. We are actually taking a quantum leap forward. For many it will feel like a far stretch from how they have been living their lives. For those who are still in denial that we need radical change and for those who are still trying to live their lives through the old paradigm, life will appear to resist them big time and it will not be pretty. What used to work is no longer working.

For those who are opening their minds to shift into a new paradigm, it is an exciting, exhilarating, and powerful time to be alive. Yes, there is much work to do but if we each play our part, it will be worth it. If every single one of us woke up and answered the call all at once, in an instant the entire world would be transformed. We have actually arrived at a time when it is easier to be awake, to live consciously than it is to be asleep at the wheel. We can't pretend, ignore, numb out, and resist like we used to. That has become too painful. We can live consciously and thrive with purpose or live unconsciously, resist life, and suffer. We each have the right to choose but the stakes are higher and the consequences are more intensely experienced.

Now let me stretch your mind a little bit more with another perspective. What if some of us have a role to play in the awakening of humanity that appears to be a negative role? What if some of us are meant to play the role of the villain or the bad guy? What if their soul has agreed they would stay asleep at the wheel in this lifetime to fulfil a role that would shake people up so much that they felt like they had no choice but to face their fears, find their voice, speak their truth, and stand in love? What if some people need to feel the ground shaking and cracking beneath their feet in order to change their ways and wake up? What if all that appears to be happening in the world today is a "collective rock bottom" forcing many people to wake up? We have only to read any daily newspaper to grasp that this could be true.

Some people still need to learn the hard way. Some people need to get the point by having their suffering bring them to their knees. Some people need to hit rock bottom and fall flat on their back before they can look up and see there is another way.

Dwight Pledger, my good friend and fellow Les Brown Platinum Speaker, always says, "When the pain of staying the same is greater than the pain of change, change is possible." For some, the world will change when the pain of its staying the same is greater than the pain of change. Many of us are feeling inspired to teach, support, empower, and inspire as many people as we possibly can to find a path of least resistance, to say YES before the resistance is so strong that they have no choice.

There is another way. It doesn't have to be so painful.

When we stop resisting life, life will stop resisting us. We need to stop saying no to what is happening and accept there is something bigger playing out. When we stop resisting, we will stop bumping up against our own fears, and our experience of life will change in an instant. When we can accept what is, embrace change, and say yes to play our part, we will discover a sense of purpose and strength that will carry us through every challenge on our path.

In the last three years in my advanced mentoring program for conscious leaders, entrepreneurs, healers, and intuitive coaches, I have seen a repeating pattern of a call for deep surrender. It was a layer of fear that needed to be healed before these leaders could step more into the expression of their gifts. I had already had to clear the same pattern within myself, and that led to my intuition becoming even more laser focused and my business expanding with ease and grace. The thick dense layer of resistances I am referring to resides in the solar plexus, the area at the upper middle part of the abdomen where the diaphragm rests. It is like a fist gripping with all its might holding on for dear life.

The words I would hear each time are "Don't make me do it. Don't make me let go." It is the last-ditch effort of the ego mind to resist life and desperately hold on to control. We are each being asked to surrender our personal will, which is based on our limited programmed mind. We are each being asked to trust our higher will, which is based on the knowing in our heart. Resistance is the gap between what our mind thinks and what our heart knows. When our mind is in alignment with our heart, there is no resistance. When our mind is not, there is resistance; the bigger the gap, the greater the experience of resistance. Many of my clients feel the calling in their heart deeply but in their mind they are afraid to fully embrace and embody their gifts. They are often afraid of judgment from others and their ego mind convinces them it is not safe so they resist. The calling in their heart keeps getting stronger and the resistance in their mind creates a bigger and bigger gap and more and more suffering. It is only when we identify the root of the resistance or the limited belief in their mind that we can close the gap of resistance and they can align with their heart.

We each need to get out of our head and into our heart and trust the guidance we will receive. Our heart holds wisdom beyond the limitations of our mind. Our heart is a bridge to our Soul and it provides us with a universal perspective that serves all of us. When we let our hearts take the lead, we will receive directions from moment to moment like a step-by-step recipe. It is our Soul speaking directly to us, guiding our every move based on what is for everyone's highest good. We each need to make a choice. We either continue to resist and say, "No, don't make me," or we choose love, we surrender, and we say YES to the path we are meant to take. When we say YES, we are saying YES to all of life and to our contribution that serves all lives everywhere all at once.

~

Our heart is a bridge to our Soul and it provides us with a universal perspective that serves all of us.

~

I invite you to drop into your body and bring your awareness to your solar plexus. Imagine opening your fist, letting go of your resistance, surrendering your fear, and allowing your heart to take the driver's seat. We let go of control and trust our intuition and then we lead with our hearts.

As we let go and trust, we can watch the resistance as it falls away in an instant and allows us to meet life in all its glory. As we each awaken to our fullest potential and extend our greatest contribution to humanity, the world will evolve in a way that will blow our minds wide open; miracles will be celebrated all around the globe.

What the world needs is for each of us to wake up fully

to be of the highest service to all of humanity leading with an open, vulnerably brave, compassionate heart. That is a choice for love each of us can make in any moment. As we stop resisting life, life will stop resisting us, and it will open each of us up to miracles that go beyond what our mind would ever think is possible. Let go, surrender your resistance, open your fist, and extend your heart to everyone. That is a true act of love we can each choose now.

Day 29

Life by Default, Life by Design, or Life by Divine

Day 29 ~
Life by Default, Life by Design, or Life by Divine

About eighty to ninety percent of the population are asleep at the wheel of life and living life by default. The other ten to twenty percent are living by design or by divine. Everyone needs to be moving with the intention to live life by divine if we are to contribute to the course correction that will uplift all of humanity.

~

People living by default are asleep at the wheel.

~

There are three ways to live life: by default, by design, or by divine. If people live by default, they are asleep at the wheel, living unconsciously, thinking they are in control, and blaming the world for all of their problems. They are living in the state of mind that life is happening to them, as I explained on Day 20 in "A Living Breathing Classroom Designed Just for You." People who are living by default are on autopilot, reacting to life, and fighting for a sense of control. They lack trust in life and live with a strong defense, always on guard and/or feeling like a victim of circumstances. Most people who live by default are driven by fear and tend to resist life, thereby creating more suffering and pain.

When someone lives by design, they are living with more awareness and they are conscious of how their response to life influences their experience of life. They recognize they are capable of designing a life that they love. They are using their mind in a more positive way and often co-creating with their heart, but they are still leading with their head. The mind still believes it is in the driver's seat; it could also be that the heart and the mind are taking turns driving. These people tend to respond to life versus reacting to it. They use life's challenges to heal their limited mind. They are in the unwinding phase of awakening and at the same time feeling a sense of control as they realize their internal world directly influences their external world. Their trust is building through each experience of manifestation and co-creation, and they are building faith in love and reacting less and less with fear.

~

People living by design tend to respond to life versus reacting to it; they are still leading with their head.

~

When someone is living life by divine, they are living with full awareness and have surrendered to allow their heart to take the lead in every moment. Waking up to this level is often a process that occurs over time and requires deep trust and blind faith. For most people, it will take time to build their confidence. They respond to life knowing there is always a bigger picture playing out, a perspective that only their heart has access to. They have surrendered their personal will for their higher will. They are deepening their connection between their heart, their soul, and the Divine (also referred to as the Higher Self, the Universe, God, Spirit, and Source). They feel a sense of purpose and they trust their life is unfolding as it is meant to. They let their heart lead and are consciously making a choice to use their life as a classroom to heal and remove all blocks to love as they align with their heart's calling.

Some people will shift back and forth between each phase, whereas others will stand solid in one before moving to another. Creating awareness about what phase you are living will empower you to make a conscious choice to shift to the one that you believe will be best for you at this time in your life. Ultimately, we are each being called to live life by Divine, but it will take some people more time to process their fears, reprogram their mind and limiting beliefs, heal their past hurts, build their trust, and let their heart take the lead. It is important to practise patience with each other, be compassionate and, at the same time, encourage others no matter what phase they are living in.

You may have a role to play in awakening others or you may not. Only your heart can lead you and unless you receive clear directions to take inspired action, you will need to mind your own business.

In my mind, I think I am fully capable and have the ability to support every single person in the world through this process, but in my heart I know I am only to support those I am meant to support. My heart leads me to those I am meant to work with, directly or indirectly, and I can look upon everyone else with love. I can see them as capable. I can see them as worthy. I can see their heart calling to them. I can trust they will hear the call or someone else will be guided to support them in divine right timing. The rest is none of my business. I can only do what I am guided to do because I live life by Divine and I follow the directions of my heart in every moment. I know the guidance that comes through my heart is serving the highest good for all of humanity, so I play my part and only my part knowing everyone is taken care of in the way they need it most.

Growing up, I spent most of my life living by default. I was asleep at the wheel doing my best to try and navigate this thing called life. It was painful and I created way more suffering for myself because everything was automatically being filtered through my limited mind with its victim mentality programming. Looking back I was really good at manifesting and making things happen, but I never thought I was making those things happen. When I set my mind to something combined with a lot of hard work, it would come together. I didn't give myself credit for anything I created because my underlying belief was that nothing I did was good enough. Not being good enough was the force that was driving me to prove my worth, excel at everything I put my energy toward, and ultimately achieve all my goals. There was a lot of blood, sweat, and tears but, in the end, nothing was ever good enough.

It wasn't until I was in my early twenties that I woke up to realize that I was actually making things happen. I realized the power of my mind and my ability to influence how my life circumstances were unfolding. As I started to challenge my own limiting thoughts, I started to feel more and more empowered. I started living life by design. My eyes were opening and I was waking up to a new way of living and responding to life. I could see the connection between my intention, my mindset, and the outcome.

I also started to see a pattern between manifesting successfully and employing self-sabotaging patterns. I would self-sabotage when I set a goal that was not in alignment with what I believed I deserved or felt worthy of. This was particularly evident when it came to money. Unwinding from my money blocks has been some of my most challenging healing work. My mind was deeply programmed for lack and limitation with a boatload of unworthiness. It was the perfect recipe for living pay cheque to pay cheque. Living life by design was amazing and empowering but still limited, because everything was filtered through my mind. On the outside I was a master manifester, but on the inside I now know I was still playing small because my mind's filter was limited and holding me back, especially around money.

In the last ten years, I have learned how to bypass my limited mind and trust my heart to lead me. I started to allow my heart to make all my decisions. A huge shift happened when I surrendered my thoughts and ideas about my gift of manifesting and allowed my heart to take the lead fully and completely. While my mind was still trying to navigate, I would find myself on occasion going between life by divine and life by design and back again to life by divine. But more often than not, I was in a place of deep surrender and trust. It was as though my Soul was guiding me from a higher perspective.

At some point, I felt a higher call to expand my Heart Led Living business and community. In the same moment that I felt a huge expansion, I felt a powerful resistance in my solar plexus. I was having some digestive issues at the time and had a partial blockage in my intestine. It was as though my guts were gripping my food, preventing it from passing through. It started to get worse and for about two years, I was eating mostly liquids because if I ate too much solid food, it was extremely painful.

My resistance was growing as I searched for answers to release this block in my intestines. I could palpate it as I pressed into my abdomen with my fingers and I could follow the shape of it. I started to call it my snake, because it was an S shape of density. Part of me just wanted the block to move and get the heck out of me, but I knew it was there to teach me something. I spent a lot of time nurturing, loving, cursing, hating, fighting, surrendering, questioning, searching, reflecting, struggling, and giving up only to surrender again, over and over again. It was an emotional roller-coaster, but all the while I knew it had something to teach me.

The strongest feeling I had was when I would tune into the vision I received from my heart about expanding my Heart Led Living Community. Instantly, my solar plexus would contract more and I would hear the words "Don't make me do it!" It was the last ditch effort of my ego mind to keep me playing small. I knew in my heart my community was meant to grow to at least a hundred members. One morning I received a vision in meditation that it was meant to grow to a thousand. That felt like a stretch for my mind, but at the same time it felt true in my heart. The resistance was strong as it came through in thoughts of fear about my health and not being able to hold space for a thousand members. Again I would feel a gripping fear and hear the words "Don't make me do it!"

I finally shed light on my biggest blind spot. It was the battle waged by my personal will, my ego's will. My ego was fighting my heart. It was resisting the call of my Soul. I was fighting and resisting the path that I knew in my heart was calling me so strongly. The contraction in my gut was me holding on for dear life to the energy of "No! Don't make me do it!" I needed to say YES to the call in my heart to expand my business.

I moved my awareness into my heart. Suddenly, I received a vision of ten thousand Heart Led Living Community members. I lost my breath for a moment.

Slowly, I invited my breath to soften and flow and the vision continued to expand. I felt enormous abundance flowing in, as well as an outward flow to support our global humanitarian work that empowers women and girls to step into their full potential. I felt the rising of a powerful force for change and I saw our hearts united in love. I softened my solar plexus and surrendered once more. The energy of YES filled every cell in my body. I felt alive with love and my entire being expanded as I heard the words "Heart YES Movement." I had a glimpse of something so much bigger than myself and, at the same time, I felt an authentic heart YES to be the gentle shepherd to allow it to come to fruition.

Ten thousand voices of hope, inspiration, and love. I suddenly saw other light leaders gathering around me. I was not alone. My entire body softened and I could feel my Soul embodiment. I could feel my heart YES. I could feel a full surrender of my ego mind and the alignment of my heart and soul with my life's calling. I had come home and I was now ready to fulfil my greatest calling and contribution to humanity. I have let go of the reigns and shifted completely into living life by divine. Once I healed the root of my resistance to expanding my life and business, my physical resistance shifted and my intestinal snake passed and my digestion improved. Peace, love, and a sense of wholeness now surround me and fill my entire being. I feel at one with everyone, everything, everywhere, all at once.

I am committed to taking my life to the next level, knowing it will have a global impact that will uplift humanity and unite us in love for each other and our planet. I know many more people are also feeling this call to shift from living life by design to living life by divine. It connects us to a realm of unlimited potential and a field of enormous possibility, because our decisions will come from a higher place and will not be filtered through our limited minds. As we allow the divine force to move through us, as us, this force will carry us, guide us, and direct us in every moment. This force is acting on behalf of everyone, everywhere, all at once, all as one. One by one we will surrender to the grand plan that is serving the highest good of all humanity as well as our planet.

Are you ready to live life by divine?

Are you willing to surrender your personal will in exchange for your higher will, your Soul's will?

Will you say YES to the calling in your heart?

Are you willing to play your part?

Will you unite your heart with ours and say YES, YES, YES?

We are all in this together. We need you. Our entire planet needs you. Just say YES, then follow your heart and watch the miracles unfold as your divine life comes to fruition. It is so worth it!

Day 30

Answering the Call for Love

Day 30 ~
Answering the Call for Love

Before you were born, a tiny seed was planted in the core of your being and the directions to achieve its full potential were placed in your heart. Let's take a look at an acorn seed. It has the potential to become a mighty oak tree as long as it is planted in fertile soil, is watered frequently, receives the rays of the sun, and is held in a nurturing environment. The seed within each of us has the potential to thrive, expand, and grow in ways we can't even begin to comprehend. The potential beauty, the abundance of miracles, and the depth of love contained within that seed are beyond what our minds can conceive.

~

We each hold within our hearts the recipe, the directions, the guidance to provide the most ideal environment to fulfil our unique gift's potential and to live out our destiny.

~

Our individual seed represents our calling, our greatest potential, our purpose, our unique gift, and our extraordinary potential. We each hold within our hearts the recipe, the directions, the guidance to provide the most ideal environment to fulfil its potential and to live out our destiny. Each seed is unique and provides everything we need to extend our greatest contribution to humanity. There is one common thread in every seed, in every living being, and that is love.

Our capacity to love deeply is inside each one of us. When we make a conscious choice to choose love, we are saying YES to the calling in our heart that has the potential to serve all of humanity directly or indirectly. One of the ten life principles in my book *Heart Led Living ~ When Hard Work Become Heart Work* is "Choose love." In every moment we have the ability to make one of two choices, love or fear. If we go a little deeper and open our minds to another perspective around fear, we can begin to recognize that fear is actually a call for love. As we shift our mindset and embrace the truth that every action or nonaction is either a choice for love or a call for love, we can answer other people's fears and their calls for love with compassion.

~

Every action and every nonaction is either a choice for love or a call for love.

~

The potential to choose love is always there within us. It is our true nature. We have been programmed to be afraid of fear, to contract, to withdraw, and to fight against life, but that only adds more fear to the recipe. In other words when we meet fear with fear, fear expands. When we can see that another's fear is simply a call for love, we can meet their fear with love and love expands.

My first visit to the Kibera Slum in Nairobi, Kenya was overwhelming; it challenged me to the core of my being. The Kibera Slum is one of the most densely populated areas of extreme poverty in the world. It is estimated that there are one million people living in one square mile of land with most of them earning less than a dollar a day.

I was directed to walk in between my two local guides so they could keep me safe.

My first steps into the slums involved stepping over the river of sewage that crosses one of the main streets. The smell was intense—it hit my nose like a wall. I had to talk myself down and focus on taking one step a time. I could feel the despair, suffering, pain, desperation, trauma, and collective emotional history coming at me from every direction like sharp thorns in my heart, mind, and body. As an empath and healer, I could feel and sense the collective emotional suffering and physical trauma in my own body. It came at me from every direction and I have never felt so much intensity concentrated in one small area. My heart became heavy with grief and I quickly felt deeply emotional.

I was relieved to step into one family's home and listen to the story of their daily challenges. There was a six-year-old girl who was curious and shy. She didn't speak English and I didn't understand Swahili, so we communicated with simple gestures, smiles, and eye contact. I reached into my bag and brought out a sticker of a butterfly. Her eyes lit up as she looked at her mom for permission to take it from me. I could feel her gratitude, and her smile grew when I placed it in her hand.

Each time I opened my bag, her eyes went wide with immense anticipation. I brought out some more stickers and a few bracelets. She was so grateful for anything I had to give. I could feel a deep connection and love extended from my heart. All my experiences of the fear, pain, and suffering disappeared in that moment and instead I felt the joy and gratitude in both our hearts for this beautiful exchange. I found peace and purpose for my visit.

When we started to make our way back out of the slums, our guide was leading us through the safest path, avoiding areas where they wouldn't be able to protect me. We were walking in between the mud homes on narrow paths with streams of sewage flowing between our steps. The smell was intense and I could feel my chest tightening with the overwhelming collective energy of suffering once again. It took all my focus just to breathe and not panic.

I could hear my ego mind taking over and bringing me down into a wormhole. "What am I doing here? I have no business being here. This is too much. I can't do this." I looked down and I stopped. My only option at this point on the path was to step directly into the stream of sewage. I looked up at my guide for another option and with a soft loving voice she said, "One step at a time." I took a deep breath and I stepped into the sewage and continued on the path.

Once we arrived back to the main road, I was at the edge of my emotional capacity. My fear was expanding as it mixed with the collective fear of many who live in the slums. I surrendered and prayed for another perspective. "Please show me another perspective, because the one I am holding is way too painful."

In that moment I could hear children chanting and singing, "How are you? How are you? How are you?" I looked around and my eyes made contact with a group of young children jumping up and down and singing to get my attention. When my eyes met theirs, they giggled and scattered like shy mice. It was the only English they knew and they were excited it got my attention. Suddenly, my eyes started to land on the children's faces as they played. They smiled and waved at me with great anticipation of getting my attention.

My heart started to expand with love as I smiled back. My eyes welled up with tears as I was moved by the children. I found joy in the middle of the Kibera Slum and all my fear and feelings of despair disappeared once again. I watched with joy in my heart as the children played with a stick, a boot, a set of wheels that had broken off a toy truck, a deflated ball; they were happy with whatever they could find. They were smiling, dancing, and singing.

I met the collective fear I felt with love and love expanded. The shift from fear to love opened my mind to see the possibilities, the potential, the love, the joy, the connection. The shift broke open my heart in a way that I can't capture in words. All I know is that I was changed at the core of my being and my fear was transformed. It took me a few days to process what I had witnessed and I started to bless the women and children in the slums. I started to see them as capable. I may not have had money to give at that time, but I had a lot of love, compassion, and healing energy to extend, and that carried me through the rest of my trip as well as through my next visit.

On my second trip to Kenya, I had no fear. It was odd at first and I would occasionally look around for it. My fear had disappeared. I walked through the streets of the slums, visiting the schools, and handing out small toy cars and trucks my son had donated with a peaceful calm and open loving heart. I was calm even when our car was surrounded by soldiers with rifles pointing at me through the window. I was deeply present and I had no fear. I heard my heart speak: "Open your window." And I calmly opened my window. Once the soldiers saw me, they lowered their rifles. I met their fear with unwavering love and they calmed down.

Upon my return to Canada I became clear that our Heart Led Living Foundation needed to be based on love. We extend love and healing energy as well as emotional and financial support to women and girls in Kenya. We do not give from a place of fear, obligation, or self-sacrifice. Anything given from fear only expands fear. We ask that donations are heart led to ensure that love is the primary energy we extend. As we meet fear with love, love expands. Never underestimate the power of a choice for love. Love is the most powerful force that exists and the potential for love is within us. It is not just in some of us; it is within all of us, every living being, without exception. The potential for love to grow, expand, and uplift humanity resides in each of our seeds. When we create a loving environment of love for self and others, and follow the unique directions to nurture the seed within our hearts, we will each grow in ways that have the potential to change the world and unify us in love.

~

Love is the most powerful force that exists and the potential for love is within us.

~

Yes, it feels like a big calling and it is indeed a big call for love, but that is what is necessary to shake us up and wake us up. The time is NOW. No more delay. We have reached the tipping point, the point of no return, the choice point where we all get to choose to answer the call for love for ourselves and for everyone, everywhere. As we continue to unite in love, we become an even more powerful force for change. The world needs all of us to unite in love.

The recipe is already within you. Your potential, your gift, your unique path to serve humanity with love are all within your own heart. As you trust your intuition, follow the directions of your unique recipe and, as you let your heart take the lead, you will become a beacon of love. No more delay. Answer the call for love within your own heart and together we can answer the call for love for all of humanity and we can become a force for change, evolution, and unity.

When we bring our hearts together and unify in love for each other and our planet, we will illuminate the path for others and together we will light up the world.

Autobiography of Sue Dumais

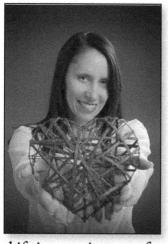

Sue Dumais is a Global Impact Visionary Leader answering the call to heal the world. She is a best-selling author, an international speaker, a divine leader of light leaders, a sacred guide, a gifted intuitive healer, a miracle weaver and a global voice of HOPE and inspiration for the "Heart YES Movement."

Sue brings the gifts of insight, awareness, and self-empowerment to her global audience creating a shift in consciousness from head to heart. Her mission is to ignite our hearts to uplift humanity and unify us in love for each other and our planet.

A humanitarian at heart, Sue created the Heart Led Living Foundation to extend love and healing energy as well as emotional and financial support to empower women and girls in Kenya.

Sue's recent book is Expect Miracles ~ 10 Beautiful Souls Share Stories of Hope, Inspiration and Transformation. Her previous book Heart Led Living ~ When Hard Work Becomes Heart Work features the ten heart led principles that are designed to help awaken our innate ability to heal, trust our intuition, lead with our heart, and discover our "YES!" for life.

Through a divine blend of transformational guidance, unique perspectives, and a radically honest approach, Sue fosters deep healing and a profound awakening. She guides others to hear, answer, and trust the highest calling of their heart. Sue is passionate about illuminating the path for others as they discover, embrace, and embody their heart YES.

Learn more at heartledliving.com

Online Programs and Resources

Join our Heart YES Movement (www.heartledliving.com)

Heart Led Living Community Membership
(www.heartledliving.com)

Intuitive Coaching Certification Program
(www.heartledliving.com)

Heart Led Business Mentoring & Mastermind for Conscious
Business Leaders, Heart-Centered Entrepreneurs, Holistic
Practitioners & Light Leaders (www.heartledliving.com)

Protecting Your Precious Energy audio program
(www.heartledliving.com)

Fertility Yoga & Meditation Kit (www.familypassages.ca)

International Fertility Yoga Teacher Training online course
(www.familypassages.ca)

Hire Sue as a Speaker

Sue Dumais blends her gifts as an intuitive healer, heart led
living coach, yoga mind body specialist and authentic story
teller to provide a transformational experience like no other.
Sue has been known to belly dance on stage bringing audiences
to their feet with tears in their eyes and joy in their hearts.

She truly owns her power on stage and has been teaching,
speaking and training for more than 20 years. Sue has been
honoured to share the stage with Dr Christiane Northrup,
Dr Denis Waitely, Marianne Williamson and Les Brown

and she has spoken in front of audiences 10,000 strong with unshakeable confidence.

Sue brings a deep level of insight, awareness and self empowerment to her audience. Her gift is to inspire other to awaken their innate ability to heal, trust their intuition, follow their hearts and discover their YES for life. To hire Sue visit www.heartledliving.com/about/speaking

Other Books

Expect Miracles ~ 10 beautiful souls share stories of Hope, Inspiration & Transformation

Heart Led Living ~ When Hard Work Becomes Heart Work

Websites

Heart Led Living: www.heartledliving.com
Family Passages: www.familypassages.ca

Social Media

Facebook: www.facebook.com/heartledliving
www.facebook.com/groups/heartyes
Twitter: www.twitter.com/heartledliving
Blog: www.heartledliving.com/blog
Instagram: www.instagram.com/suedumais/
Pinterest: pinterest.com/suedumais/boards
YouTube: https://www.youtube.com/user/SueDumais
LinkedIn: www.linkedin.com/in/sue-dumais-0851231/